FIT SOUL

TOOLS, TACTICS & HABITS FOR OPTIMIZING

SPIRITUAL FITNESS

by

BEN GREENFIELD

TABLE OF
CONTENTS

WHO AM I?

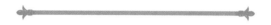

I got lucky.

On second thought, I need to work that "lucky" expression out of my vernacular. I still find myself lazily using it, even when writing. Luck, coincidence and seeming serendipity are all simply signs of a great God doing His work in mysterious ways.

A more appropriate phrase would be *"God blessed me."*.

Why do I say this?

Frankly, I was born into a very happy, stable home. The second-spawned of five siblings (one older brother, one younger brother and two younger sisters), I was raised and homeschooled by newly Christian parents who - after moving to North Idaho to escape sin, drugs, crime and turmoil in their cities of Miami (father) and Detroit (mother) - had a deep yearning in their hearts to raise their children in a safe, protected and spiritually nourishing environment steeped in deep love and connection.

So as a result, from the very beginning, I didn't really have any "childhood trauma." I experienced very little adolescent angst. I was perfectly happy spending my days with my nose in a book, a violin on my shoulder, a chess pawn in my fingers and a basketball or tennis racquet in my hands. Don't get me wrong: my childhood wasn't plain-jane or ho-hum, but did indeed involve very little drama, fights, heartache or trouble. No drugs. No alcohol. No social media drama (heck, no smartphones!). Tons of reading. Very little pop culture drivel. Plenty of church and Sunday School. You get the idea.

Here's a perfect illustrative example: I recently came across a newspaper interview with me that took place when I was 14 years old. As you can see from the clipping below, the reporter astutely and accurately commented, *"the most important things in Ben's life are his God and his family..."*.

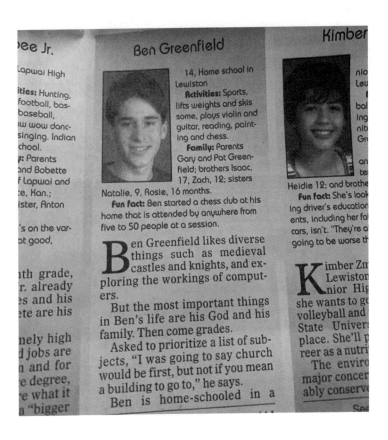

That's just how I was.

I wasn't perfect, but in most respects, I was a pretty decent kid. I loved God, I dug morality and fairness and I loved to make everybody around me happy.

THE SLIDE TO INAUTHENTICITY

But eventually, I was traumatized - that is, if you consider trauma to be defined as Dr. Gabor Mate describes it: "a loss of connection to one's true self."

See, I began college as an immature 15 year old who probably should have been more socially responsible and spiritually prepared before diving headfirst into a giant booze-infused "academic gathering" of peers to impress. Almost immediately, I began transforming myself into who I thought the world expected me to be, what folks around me perceived as cool, and anything but my true, authentic self. After all, what cool person could possibly be impressed by a homeschooled, chess-playing, fantasy-fiction-loving, Bible-believing, classical music enthusiast?

I began drinking and partying multiple times per week.

Sleeping around and treating women like objects.

Remodeling myself as a loud, boisterous, muscle-bound jock, while sidelining any of my creative or seemingly meek character traits.

Falling away from reading my Bible, praying, regularly attending church, and maintaining any semblance of union with God.

While still calling myself a Christian, my lifestyle reflected anything but. Perhaps my only saving grace - despite my pure neglect of spiritual disciplines - was that I did not shirk my academic and career disciplines during this time, and thus rose to the top of nearly every class in which I enrolled. I completed a full pre-med curriculum and attained a master's degree in exercise physiology and biomechanics, all while simultaneously moonlighting as a personal trainer, sports camp and tennis instructor, coffeeshop barista and bartender.

In my senior year of college, I married a wonderful, faithful, beautiful Christian girl named Jessa. Upon becoming a husband, I gained a slight sense of greater responsibility. I straightened up just a bit, or at least quit partying and drinking quite so much. I began to attend church more frequently, mostly to make my wife happy, but also because I had a slight stirring in my soul that it was probably the "right thing to do." Then, three years into our marriage, Jessa and I were blessed with twin boys, and my sense of responsibility even more dramatically shifted. I started a family constitution, a trust, a living will, and an investment portfolio. An outside observer may have assumed I was finally becoming a "man," though I was still an irresponsible, selfish boy on the inside.

My neglect of the spiritual disciplines was still painfully glaring. Studying Scripture, praying, meditating, fasting, silence, presence, and true worship of God were all shoved to the side in favor of pumping iron, drinking protein shakes, flexing, building a business, making money, seeking praise of men and women, and ultimately, serving my false self while simultaneously staying severely disconnected from my true self.

Often to the neglect of my young family, I began a slow slide into the escape I could afford through workaholism. I built a successful chain of personal training studios and gyms, began making six figures a year as a health and exercise junkie "guru," was nominated as America's top personal trainer, appeared on the cover of multiple fitness magazines and simultaneously rose to the peak of athletic success as an adventure athlete who hopped on planes multiple times a week to leave town and compete, an Ironman racer who trained for hours a day while my family played alone at home, and a ripped, fit, picture-perfect image of all the shallow, pleasures of the flesh that the world holds dear. My dear wife, Jessa, patiently put up with my gallivanting about the globe engaged in my pursuit of ego-inflating enjoyments. She prayed earnestly for me, did the lion's share of raising our boys, attended church by herself as I traveled nearly every Sunday, and - by the grace of God - she somehow patiently put up with being married to the spiritual equivalent of an irresponsible, selfish brat.

I bought a condo. Then a house. Then another house. A couple nice cars. Biohacking toys. More fitness equipment. Rifles, pistols, bows, arrows, spearfishing guns, gold, silver, bitcoin, and plenty of ribeye steaks. A guitar. A ukulele. A few drums. Nice things for my wife. Toys, toys and more toys for my boys. A massive library of books. A thriving nutrition supplements company. A lucrative speaking and writing career. Then finally, a dream home on ten acres of forested land in Washington state. Fame, power, money, belongings and social media followers were my holy metrics of success.

Yet even then, ten years into marriage, saturated with all the worldly success that society places on a pedestal, and from an outsider's perspective, becoming a man who had "made it" with a beautiful family, a successful career, social media fame and a fit body, I was severely broken and unhappy.

There was never enough to satisfy my carnal cravings.

I succumbed to nearly every temptation the world threw at me.

I sacrificed relationships, friends and family for all the notoriety, wealth and prosperity I thought would make me happy.

I escaped the constant pricking of my conscience with what I knew deep down to be true and right by running physically and running emotionally - filling my life with a

constant buzz of doing, doing and doing that kept me from confronting the gaping
hole of personal emptiness and unhappiness inside me.

I was disconnected from my true self.

I was traumatized without even knowing it.

And perhaps most sadly, I was disconnected from God.

My God-Shaped Hole

There was a distinct moment when I came to the realization that my priorities in life needed to seriously change and my path to the top of the mountain was in truth plunging my life, my family and relationship with God to the bottom of a dark valley.

That moment occurred when I realized I could no longer hide my rotten habits away from my patient and long-suffering wife. Upon returning from a long, solitary walk on a Sunday afternoon, I was convicted by God and broke down in front of Jessa, confessing to her that I had not been a faithful husband. Of course, I had amassed many other wrongdoings related to my inherent selfishness, but I knew that unfaithfulness to my wife was what was really eating me up from the inside out.

It was one of the most difficult conversations I've ever had. In an act of pure grace, kindness and love, Jessa forgave me, but she was hurt to the core, and for weeks our relationship, already built upon the frail foundation of an absent husband and father, became even more rocky and precarious. I feared that I had screwed everything up - big time - and that the family I loved so much was now going to be torn apart in a public and embarrassing fashion. In the later years of their marriage, I had witnessed my own parents' painful divorce, felt as though the same tragedy was about to happen in my marriage - and worse yet, I knew it was all my fault.

And so one morning, days after my confession and sitting alone in my kitchen sipping coffee while staring off into the hills behind the house in the throes of frustration, fear, shame and emotional alienation from Jessa, I realized that if I did not begin to tend to my spiritual health and restore my union with God, I really was going to lose all that really mattered in life. I was, as Mark 8:36 alludes to, going to be a man who had gained the whole world, yet lost his own soul.

That very morning, I went upstairs to the bedroom, found my dusty, neglected Bible, and cracked it open. It had been so long since I'd read God's word that I simply began with the very first chapter of Genesis.

After reading, I turned to God and began to pray. It felt awkward, foreign and strange to be speaking to the Creator whom I had neglected for so long, but I poured my heart out to Him nonetheless in a desperate cry for help and direction. Later that week, I even wrote a personal prayer and began to recite it each and every morning, a prayer I continue to recite to this very day:

"Our Father in heaven, I surrender all to you
Turn me into the father and husband you
would have for me to be
Into a man who will fulfill your great commission
And remove from me all judgment of others
Grant me your heavenly wisdom
Remove from me my worldly temptations
Teach me to listen to your still, small voice in the silence
And fill me with your peace, your love, and your joy.
Amen."

I also began to meditate.

And to journal.

As the months proceeded, I dove into the spiritual disciplines that I discuss here, voraciously consuming titles such as *Celebration of Discipline: The Path to Spiritual Growth* by Richard Foster, *Spiritual Disciplines for the Christian Life* by Donald S. Whitney, the *Spiritual Disciplines Handbook* by Adele A. Calhoun, and many other books far outside the realm of the fitness, science, nutrition and biohacking literature I'd so myopically immersed myself in for oh-too-long.

I ferociously committed myself to my family, for the first time in years learning to be fully present with my wife and twin boys, trusting on God to provide for my needs rather than engaging in frantic, desperate workaholism, and being the father, the leader and the man who I knew from my childhood that God called me to be (despite my decades-long resistance to accepting that calling and forsaking all my irresponsible boyish escapades).

Perhaps most importantly, over the next several months, God slowly opened my eyes and I began to realize that no amount of money, fame and famous friends, business success, fitness, dietary perfection, supplements, drugs, books, toys, musical instruments can fill the "God-shaped hole" within one's heart.

See, every person has a void in their life that can only be filled by God.

This God-shaped hole is simply the innate longing of the heart for something outside itself, something transcendent, something "other" and something "greater". Ecclesiastes 3:11 refers to this as the "eternity in man's heart". God made us for an eternal purpose, and only God can fulfill that deep-rooted desire for eternity. Nearly every religion that exists is based upon this innate desire to connect with someone or something greater than ourselves, and this desire can only be filled by God.

The problem is we silly, selfish humans can spend much of our life - or worse, all of our life - ignoring this hole or attempting to fill it with anything other than God. If it promises to fulfill our longing for meaning, whether business, family, sports and other hobbies, food, drink, exercise and the like, then we keep dumping it into that hole, expecting that at some point, the hole will be full and the result will be the happiness we have been craving that nothing else seems to provide. Yet by pursuing these things that are not eternal, we remain unfulfilled and continue to wonder why our lives never seem satisfactory. Sure, we can achieve happiness for a short period of time, such as when we finally get to the body fat percentage we desire, discover the perfect diet, graduate college or graduate college again, cross the finish line of a triathlon, get married and have kids, win the lottery or achieve massive business success - *but nothing fulfills the longing for eternity.*

People pursuing all things except God can certainly achieve some measure of "happiness" for a short period of time. But consider the words of King Solomon, who had all the riches, success and power one could ever wish for—in short, a vast world of wealth that many humans spend their entire lives seeking. Yet Solomon called this all dissatisfactory vanity (Ecclesiastes 1). Solomon at least realized that all worldly pleasures in the absence of God are vain. Many other rich and successful people don't even arrive at that realization. Simply consider the Hollywood suicides of individuals like Robin Williams and Marilyn Monroe, the seeming unhappiness and unfulfilled attitude of great athletes like Tiger Woods and Michael Jordan, and the wealthy, successful yet miserable status of America's dream job elite highlighted in a recent New York Times article I read on those haunting the halls at corporations such as McKinsey & Company, Google, Goldman Sachs and Apple.

Things get even worse if you, like me, are "driven," as Dr. Doug Brackman highlights so well in his book by the same name. Many of us are born with a natural genetic drive often seen in entrepreneurs, pro-athletes, inventors, adventurers, and Navy SEALs. Due to our built-in DNA hardwiring, we tend to seek thrills, success, achievement and adventure even more than the average human, resulting in rampant impulsivity, distraction, havoc, stress and diagnoses of "medical conditions" such as ADHD, ADD, or OCD. As Doug discussed when I interviewed him for my podcast, we, driven people, fight a constant lifetime uphill battle in quest for happiness until we find God, and in many cases our God-shaped hole can be an even deeper and more problematic abyss. IF this sounds familiar to you, you should read Doug's book or listen to my podcast with him (incidentally, whenever I mention a book or podcast throughout this book, I will link to it on the references page for each chapter, which is available by accessing the link at the end of each chapter - in this case *FitSoulBook.com/Introduction*.

No Regrets, Only Gratefulness

Ultimately, in the same way a square peg cannot fill a round hole, the God-shaped hole inside each of us cannot be filled by anyone or anything other than God. Not only did I eventually come to the profound realization that my own hole had been empty for a very long time, but the same was also true for my thousands upon thousands of followers in the physical culture, fitness and health world who had a similar deep, unhappy gnawing in their soul, and were craving the answers I was suddenly finding.

Now, at this point in my life, I could have had many regrets.

Regrets at having played a large part in giving many people the false impression that they could find their happiness through exercise and dieting.

Regrets at having spent so many years neglecting my own spiritual fitness while simultaneously spending inordinate amounts of time honing physical and mental fitness perfection.

Regrets that I had stepped onto so many hundreds of stages and in front of so many microphones teaching people how to satisfy their fleshly pursuits while simultaneously presenting a skewed reality of what is truly important in life.

Yet, upon reflecting upon the plan that God manifested in my life, I realized that there was no need for regret. Instead, I was washed over with the understanding that over twenty years of building a giant fitness empire, God had blessed me with a sizeable audience of people hungry for and craving the same fulfillment I had finally found. As a matter of fact, here's a snippet of a journal entry of mine from November 30, 2019, during which I was meditating upon this very concept and experiencing a temptation to be regretful of squandering years:

"...you idiot! Can't you see all along that it is a journey of no regrets, and only gratefulness? Are you ashamed of being a bright and shiny spandex gold-tan Gold's Gym Nautilus spinning As-Seen-On-TV glittery Jamba Juice fitness icon? Well DON'T BE! Why? Because look where it somehow brought you: a following, a stage, a rabid fanbase of listeners and followers who are ... get this ... all suddenly looking for answers and POP! You're the dude standing in front of them and you're standing there with the elixir in your hand and the spark in your soul. Do you really think they WANT another longevity hack or pill to pop or new dumbbell move? NO! They *THINK* that's what they want and that's certainly the shiny penny that got them to grab a ticket to the experience that is YOU, but you know what - they're now sitting on that chair, you're now standing on that stage and you've got a giant audience ready to hear what they really NEED to hear - the message of light and love and hope and fulfillment that only GOD can bring."

Yes, God works in mysterious ways. He draws straight paths with crooked lines. His path to the top of the mountain is a zig-zagging goat trail that eventually - if you listen to His voice and pray for wisdom and discernment - takes you exactly to where He desires for you to make maximum impact with the life, the purpose and the unique skillset you've been blessed with (a wonderful book that explores this "path up the mountain" concept even more fully is *The Second Mountain* by David Brooks).

THE GREAT COMMISSION

After turning to God to fill the abyss in my soul, beginning to pursue the spiritual disciplines with the same fervor as I'd been pursuing the physical disciplines, and experiencing the incredibly blessed sensation of waking each morning with a satisfied smile on face, a happy and connected family, and an extraordinary fulfillment of daily union with God, life became absolutely magical - and continues to grow more magical each day as I seek wisdom, discernment and direction from God.

But I'd be remiss not to mention another meaningful moment that occurred along the way. Five years into my journey of blissful connection to faith and family, the spark lit within my spirit burst into an absolute wildfire-like inferno when I emerged from an intense plant medicine ceremony that I had prepared for with weeks of prayer, fasting, meditation and intense focus upon my relationship with God. My intention for the plant medicine was to "turn off" my analytical brain and creatively develop a few new personal and business ideas for fully manifesting my purpose in life and impact on the world.

Wait! What's the deal with "plant medicine"?

In summary, as I also write in Chapter 20...

> *"...I certainly think that there is an appropriate, responsible and purposeful use God intended for plant (or synthetic) medicine in the very same way there is an appropriate, responsible and purposeful use for a nice Bordeaux, a touch of tobacco from a cigar or pipe, or a double espresso shot pumpkin spiced latte. For example, I personally derive a great deal of energetic and creative benefit from the left and right merging of the brain hemispheres, the increase in sensory perception, and the neuronal growth that occurs when I microdose with a bit of psilocybin or LSD on a long writing day; the relaxing or the socially and sexually enhancing benefits of a touch of MDMA or cannabis; and even the enormous spectrum of insights and ideas I gain from a more intensive so-called "journey". Plant medicine, when used responsibly, can be a blessing - but, just like alcohol, nicotine, caffeine, St. John's wort or any other popular substance humankind has discovered to adjust dials in the brain - can also be used as an addiction, an escape and a dangerous replacement for God."*

In this specific case, during twenty-seven hours of "journeying" under the guidance of a trained Christian facilitator, I was completely astonished by the fact that I did not experience a single business insight, strategic plan for my company or brand, or a host of new ideas for work and life projects.

Instead, I spent the entire session repeatedly spellbound with intense and overwhelming visualizations of the entire story of Jesus playing over and over again in intense detail: his deity, his death, his burial and his resurrection.

I spent the medicine journey dwelling upon Jesus' Hero's Journey, including all the intensity of his suffering that I write about in Chapter 9, along with the glorious message of salvation, opportunity for all of humankind to release their burdens, sin and shame, and ultimate, free solution to all of our struggles both great and small. Upon emerging from the ceremony, I knew beyond a shadow of a doubt in my heart that I must spend the rest of my life shouting this good news of deliverance from the rooftops. As a matter of fact, here's just a small snippet of the many journal entries that I logged for days after the ceremony:

> "...we can all be saved. All our sins can be washed away until we are as white as snow. All the shame that's carried in individuals and even in families for generations upon generations for thousands of years - that it is all covered by Christ, and through him, we can all be forgiven. Sure, you can keep coming back to the same old wounds over and over and over again, like a nightmarish dream. But I can tell you that unless you know that it is all covered by Christ, you will never emerge from a cycle of trauma, sin or shame. So what do you do, Ben? You armor yourself with the full armor of God. You build your soul with the spiritual disciplines. You help your children put their armor on. You help them build their spiritual disciplines. You pray. You meditate. You memorize Scripture. You go to church. You build a community. You equip spirits. You show the world yourself and your family as a living, breathing example of God's light and love. You shout this message of salvation from the rooftops until your very last dying breath, because the world needs to hear it so desperately..."

Did I need plant medicine to come fully to this realization? I doubt it. I firmly believe that some are called and some are not to that type of approach. But it certainly accelerated, in a very dramatic fashion, my awakening to the meaning and magnitude of my true calling: to use my unique purpose statement to fulfill the great commission in each and every last aspect of my life.

And what is that commission? You can find it by opening your Bible to Matthew 28:17-20, where Jesus says:

"All authority in heaven and on earth has been given to me. Go therefore and make disciples of all nations, baptizing them in the name of the Father and of the Son and of the Holy Spirit, teaching them to observe all that I have commanded you. And behold, I am with you always, to the end of the age."

We are each called, in our own unique way, to fulfill that commission. I recently discovered a good perspective on unique calling presented by Sadhu Sundur Singh, a remarkable Indian disciple of Jesus Christ (it is well worth reading his biography, linked to on the resources page for this chapter). He writes in his inspiring book *With & Without Christ*:

> *"Everyone should follow his calling and carry out his work according to his God-given gifts and capacities. The same breath is blown into flute, cornet and bagpipe, but different music is produced according to different instruments. In the same way the one spirit works in us, God's children, but different results are produced, and God is glorified through them according to each one's temperament and personality."*

I challenge you too to dwell upon what kind of instrument God made you to be and how His breath of life can fuel your unique purpose in life. Let those things that come easy to you: such as reading, teaching, speaking, art, music, crafting things with your hands, or anything else be the things that you minister to the world with - and to never feel guilty if it "comes easy." A violin can spend its entire life glancing with covetousness at a piano while wishing it could and attempting to make keyboard sounds, or that same violin could spend its life playing a beautiful, enchanting concerto that displays its full violin glory.

In Zechariah 9:9-17, you can read how God shot Israel like a lightning bolt from his battle bow. But we are all God's children, and the Bible tells us that children are like arrows in one's quiver. So also imagine that each day, God is plucking you from His mighty quiver and shooting you from His bow like a lightning bolt into the world. So where is God aiming you? Are you prepared to fly like a fiery arrow wherever He aims and calls you? That is enough about life's purpose for now, but I will return to it in detail in Chapter 8.

FORGIVENESS

These days, does my life still involve daily struggles accompanied by temptations, failures and setbacks?

You bet.

As Romans 8 (one of my favorite passages in all of Scripture) states...

...all creation groans.

> *"For the creation waits with eager longing for the revealing of the children of God; for the creation was subjected to futility, not of its own will but by the will of the one who subjected it, in hope that the creation itself will be set free from its bondage to decay and will obtain the freedom of the glory of the children of God. We know that the whole creation has been groaning in labor pains until now; and not only the creation, but we ourselves, who have the first fruits of the Spirit, groan inwardly while we wait for adoption, the redemption of our bodies."*

That's right: life will be tough and full of temptation, toil and often unpleasant work by the sweat and occasional blood of our brow. We will experience disappointments, emotional ups and downs, conflicts, turmoil and unexpected, sometimes troubling twists and turns. This will continue until the very last day we are swept into Heaven.

Furthermore, one doesn't just believe upon the Hero's Journey I describe here, then wistfully waltz off into the sunset whistling a happy tune as all of life instantly becomes magical. It takes a bit more than that. It takes a release of shame of what you have done or experienced in your life thus far, and a full casting of those concerns and burdens upon God. It also takes forgiveness, a concept perfectly illustrated in the story of Louis Zamperini, the Olympic athlete and airman who endured twenty-six torturous months in a Japanese prisoner-of-war camp, a stupendous story now illustrated fully in the book and movie *Unbroken*.

Hailed as a hero for his incredible story of survival, Zamperini, for years after his release, was emotionally scarred, filled with hatred and plagued by nightmares. He became an alcoholic, abused his wife, and neglected his young daughter. Eventually, in an act of great desperation, he attended a Billy Graham crusade, confessed his sins, entered into union with God, put his faith in Christ, experienced forgiveness and was finally delivered from his nightmarish existence. He wrote:

> *"Deciding to devote your life to God doesn't mean instantaneous, nonstop happiness. Hard work lay ahead. I fought despondency and doubt, and tried to come to terms with what had happened to me...the hardest thing in life is to forgive...forgiveness is healing."*

Zamperini's epic survival story didn't buy him happiness. It was only the grace of Jesus that filled the hole in his heart and gave him the peace and happiness he had been seeking for long. So you too (as I did) must forgive yourself and release all feelings of shame to God, ask for forgiveness from others (as I also did) for rotten things you've done in the past, and finally, as Zamperini did to his Japanese wartime tormentors, forgive others who have wronged you and who you may hold bitterness against. That is, when filled with a belief and faith in the Hero's Journey, you will embody the powerful words of 2 Corinthians 5:17:

"If anyone is in Christ, he is a new creation. The old has passed away; behold the new has come."

SUMMARY

So there you have it.

That is who I am: a new creation with a renewed and fantastically exciting lease on life.

That is also why, over the past several years, if you are a regular reader of mine you may have noticed a shift in my writing towards a less myopic focus on physical and mental fitness, and instead a more broad and necessary focus on the inclusion of spiritual fitness.

Ultimately, I am overjoyed and inspired with the clarity of life purpose I experience each day. I have, by God's mercy, been plucked from sin to salvation and from meaninglessness to purposefulness. Within this book are some of the biggest lessons

I've learned along the way.

And where do you and I go from here? I will personally continue to live out my life's purpose, which is...

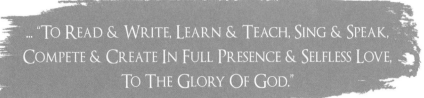

... "To Read & Write, Learn & Teach, Sing & Speak, Compete & Create In Full Presence & Selfless Love, To The Glory Of God."

This will include me not only continuing to teach you about how to care for your body and brain using the latest research, ancestral wisdom and modern science so that you too can be fully equipped to live out your own purpose in life, but also me continuing to transform (as God works in me and through me) from an adventurous boy to a more responsible and mature mentor and sage who can teach you how to not make the same mistakes I have, and who can also teach you how to tend for the one part of you that needs care and attention the most: your soul.

It is my hope and prayer that I can, within the pages of this book, help you attain not just a fit body and a fit mind but also...

...a fit soul.

This book, which began as a series of weekly "Sabbath Ramblings" on my website at BenGreenfieldFitness.com, a series which subsequently underwent significant editing and modifications, then was combined with additions from spiritual material in cut and edited sections of my book Boundless, now exists as what you are reading today - a collection of what I would consider to be my most important research, advice and wisdom on how to attain - as the title of this book implies - a Fit Soul.

Finally, to get the very most out of your Fit Soul experience, I recommend that you:

- *Read each chapter sequentially. As you finish each chapter, the skills, knowledge and insight you receive in that chapter will carry forward into subsequent chapters, gradually building your spiritual muscles as you progress through the book. In other words, I don't recommend you just flip to the middle of this book and begin with a 600 pound barbell squat. I actually wrote the chapters in this* book to be read in the specific order in which they are ordered;

- Consider reading no more than one chapter in a single sitting. Yes, each chapter is relatively short and straightforward, and if you're anything like me, you may be tempted to "powerthrough" this entire book in a day (or two, or a week) but I recommend that you dwell upon the lesson you learn in each chapter, sleep on it or walk on it to cement the lesson integration into your subconscious mind, and wait to tackle the next chapter until at least the following day;

- If you're reading the hard copy version, equip yourself with a pen or highlighter, and if the electronic version, use the handy highlight function on your e-reader and save/share insights that you find. I personally find that while I rarely have the time to re-read entire books, I do quite frequently go back and re-read all my most important highlights or folded over pages and circled or underlined passages from my favorite books, very similar to how I'll frequently return to a favorite restaurant to choose what I know is my top selected dish from that restaurant. Consider your personal highlights to be your dark chocolate soufflés, unique, aromatic cocktails and succulent meat dishes of a spiritual smorgasbord. Or, your superfood protein shakes, if you're that type of foodie. Those snacks will keep feeding your soul every time you come back to them.

Phew! I think that's enough tips. So now, where do we begin?

Let's start by ensuring you begin your journey to a fit soul with a clean slate by releasing all attachments. You're about to discover how to do just that.

For resources, references, links and additional reading and listening material for this chapter, visit FitSoulBook.com/Introduction.

CHAPTER I

FIT FOR DETACHMENT

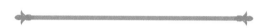

Let's talk attachments.

The world in which I spend much of my time, full of fitness junkies, exercise enthusiasts, biohackers and healthy living zealots, tends to be pretty darn attached.

Attached to our perfectly comprised meals, pantry and kitchen. God forbid we swing open the refrigerator door and not have enough organic stevia for our superfood smoothie.

Attached to our daily exercise session, so much that we can feel guilty, unhappy or even mildly depressed if we must take a walk in the sunshine because of a tweaked shoulder that makes us miss the gym.

Attached to the wearable that magically tells us whether we are rested and ready for the day or whether we had a bad night of sleep, no matter how we actually feel. Data doesn't lie, right?

Yep, we're the ones making a mad scramble in a hotel room to find something to prop our feet up on for our morning poop because the Marriott doesn't have squatty potty stools, ripping sheets off the bed to make blackout curtains to remove every sliver of light at night, and wandering around the gym looking for the vibration platform, ketone esters and blood flow restriction bands because that's what we need for a good workout.

We're the ones who go on a camping trip with fifteen extra pounds of gear: our supplements, our noise blocking headphones, our special sleeping pillow and our miniature infrared light device.

We're the ones heading out to the restaurant with our special back-up healthy sea salt and extra virgin olive oil so we can eat just like we do back home.

Perhaps you aren't part of this extreme health enthusiast world, and you're chuckling at this seeming ridiculousness. But we are all attached to many, many objects and pursuits. Perhaps they're not "healthy things" per se. You can be attached to wine and weed, coffee and energy drinks, epic vacations and adventures, cars, boats, homes, gardens, pets, shoes, or even just your favorite coat.

But can you and I release those attachments?

Are all these attachments in life weighing you down, keeping you chained and distracting you from being fully satisfied with the immense beauty of simplicity? Or are you able to view them as simply pleasures, comforts and blessings from God that you've perhaps grown to become attached to?

Your body.

Your biohacks.

Money.

Drugs and supplements and microdoses.

Food.

Knowledge. Podcasts. Books.

The social media feed and direct messages check-in.

Can you look at any of these and, as Anthony De Mello says in his book *Awareness*:

> "I really do not need you to be happy. I'm only deluding myself in the belief that without you I will not be happy. But I really don't need you for my happiness; I can be happy without you. You are not my happiness, you are not my joy."

I challenge you this week to say that statement to anything and everything you're attached to. Verbally, aloud and enthusiastically. Memorize this statement if you must. I did, then I spent a month practicing saying this phrase - even to my morning cup of coffee - and it was quite powerful and eye-opening.

As you begin this practice, also consider the following: *in the same way that it is not within your human power to resist every last temptation that this world throws at you, it is also not within your human power to fully detach from anything in life.* To experience both resistance to temptation and release from attachments, you must rely upon the power that God bestows upon you.

For example, John 8:32 tells us that *we shall know the truth, and the truth shall set us free.*

1 Corinthians 10:13 reads, *"There hath no temptation taken you but such as is common to man: but God is faithful, who will not suffer you to be tempted above that ye are able; but will with the temptation also make a way to escape, that ye may be able to bear it."*

Jesus' prayer in Matthew 6:13 finishes with a call to *"...lead us not into temptation, but deliver us from evil: For thine is the kingdom, and the power, and the glory, for ever. Amen."*

Collectively, from these three anecdotes of Scripture, I can clearly identify two ways that we can be empowered to release attachments to anything in life: 1) immersing ourselves in truth, particularly by reading and hearing the absolute truth of the Bible each day and 2) praying earnestly to God each day for resistance to temptations, and in the case of attachments, praying for a way of escape from that attachment.

So in summary, Anthony Di Mello's quote should always also be accompanied with daily immersion in Scripture, along with a prayer to God that he would empower us to release whatever attachments we happen to be experiencing in our daily life.

Finally, in Ecclesiastes 1:2-9, you can read the words of King Solomon, a man who "had it all":

> *"Vanity of vanities," says the Preacher; "Vanity of vanities, all is vanity." What profit has a man from all his labor in which he toils under the sun? One generation passes away, and another generation comes; But the earth abides forever. The sun also rises, and the sun goes down and hastens to the place where it arose. The wind goes toward the south, and turns around to the north; the wind whirls about continually and comes again on its circuit. All the rivers run into the sea, yet the sea is not full; to the place from which the rivers come, there they return again. All things are full of labor; man cannot express it. The eye is not satisfied with seeing, nor the ear filled with hearing. That which has been is what will be, that which is done is what will be done. And there is nothing new under the sun."*

Here is a man to whom God gave everything. Yet he knew that, despite our never-ending search for belongings, pleasures, wealth, power, status, and materialistic goods, everything in the absence of God is all vanity that eventually slips away like wind blowing through the desert sand. Perhaps this is why it is so hard for those who pursue their precious attachments as their primary priority in life find it so difficult to discover the eternal happiness that comes from God.

The "rich young ruler" in Mark 10:17-30 is the penultimate example of this difficulty:

> *"Jesus was setting out on a journey when a man ran up, knelt before him and put this question to him, 'Good master, what must I do to inherit eternal life?' Jesus said to him, 'Why do you call me good? No one is good but God alone. You know the commandments: You must not kill; You must not commit adultery; You must not steal; You must not bring false witness; You must not defraud; Honour your father and mother.' And he said to him, 'Master, I have kept all these from my earliest days.' Jesus looked steadily at him and loved him, and he said, 'There is one thing you lack. Go and sell everything you own and give the money to the poor, and you will have treasure in heaven; then come, follow me.' But his face fell at these words and he went away sad, for he was a man of great wealth."*

Sound familiar? I'll hazard a guess that the rich young ruler could very well have frittered away the remainder of his short life on this earth continually seeking more and more to fill his God-shaped hole in his soul, and may have unhappily passed away on a couch of plush cushions in a giant mansion somewhere. Sadly, he was not fit to detach.

Are you?

In the book *Absolute Surrender*, you can find the first step to become fit enough to surrender everything to God, including your attachments. Here is what author Andrew Murray writes in that book:

> *"You may be a very earnest, godly, devoted believer, in whom the power of the flesh is still very strong. That is a very solemn truth. Peter, before he denied Christ, had cast out devils and had healed the sick. Yet, the flesh had power; and, the flesh had room in him. Oh, beloved, we have to realize that it is because there is so much of that*

self-life in us that the power of God cannot work in us as mightily as He desires that it should work. Do you realize that the great God is longing to double His blessing, to give tenfold blessing through us? But there is something hindering Him, and that something is a proof of nothing but the self-life. We talk about the pride of Peter, and the impetuosity of Peter, and the self-confidence of Peter. It is all rooted in that one word, self Christ had said, "Deny self," and Peter had never understood, and never obeyed. Every failing came out of that."

But Andrew goes on to explain that there was the turning point in the life of Peter. Christ had said to him: "You cannot follow me now" (John 13:36). Peter was not in a "fit state" to follow Christ, because he had not yet fully given himself up for Christ. But when he went out and wept bitterly, then came a great change. Christ previously said to him: "When thou art converted, strengthen thy brethren." (Luke 22:32). At this point, after weeping and giving everything up to Jesus, Peter was surrendered, converted from self and free from attachments to rise to his true calling and to fully understand what was truly important in life.

You might be thinking...

...that is the problem with me; it is always the self-life, self-comfort, self-consciousness, self-pleasing, and self will that keeps me from giving up all my attachments.

So how are you to get rid of all the "selfish self" thoughts? It is only by surrendering all to God and fully following Jesus that you can rid yourself of attachments. Nothing else can give deliverance from the power of self. And what does He ask you to do?

Luke 9:23 is quite clear: *"If anyone would come after me, let him deny himself and take up his cross daily and follow me"*.

Once again, I ask you: are you fit enough to detach, to deny self and to take up your cross daily? If you find yourself struggling with releasing attachments, it can often help to become more self-aware of your decisions, your thought patterns and most importantly, your presence. In the next chapter, you'll learn how.

For resources, references, links and additional reading and listening material for this chapter, visit FitSoulBook.com/Chapter1.

CHAPTER II

THE BREASTPLATE OF PRESENCE

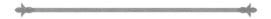

On a Sunday night last year, during a long meditation and breathwork session, God anointed me with His Presence. It came out of the blue. I was never really fully aware of how unpresent, constantly busy and distracted I am and have grown to be for so long until He spoke this truth to me in a moment of silence.

It began with me meditating upon the way I spend my day, and dwelling upon the Groundhog-day-esque nature of much of my life at that time: accomplish one task, move on to the next task, complete the next piece of content, read the next book, listen to the next podcast, prepare for the next meal, have "quick conversations" on the phone, shoot off hurried email replies, do a workout, eat dinner, spend an often rushed evening with the family, rinse, wash and repeat.

But see, God cares about each day. Sure, 2 Peter 3:8 in the Bible says that a thousand years are as a single day to God, yet this doesn't mean he doesn't still care for each of these days, hours, minutes, seconds, and microseconds.

And this means that for us to be fully grateful, fully aware, fully impactful, fully purposeful, fully excellent, and fully living to the glory of God we must also be present each day, present each hour, present each minute, present each second, present each microsecond, and perhaps most importantly: present each breath.

This anointing of an extreme awareness of Presence that God gifted to me is hard to describe, but I will try. I visualized and felt Presence fitted upon my torso, almost like the most thin, delicate, fragile glass breastplate you can imagine. It was (and is, as I visualize it even now) completely translucent, shimmering, glowing, and flowing with each twist and turn of my body. Like glass, Presence can be shattered at a moment's notice, but unlike glass—and more like water or gel or some other seamless fluid—it can instantly reform after it is broken, as long as the awareness of the broken Presence and the desire for restored Presence returns. As one learns to care for this "breastplate of Presence," one can grow better and better at keeping it from shattering, and reforming it when it is broken.

One of the best ways to maintain the integrity of Presence is with your breath. Imagine that each of your inhales charges your Presence with a deep white and blue light, and each exhale sends tendrils, vibrations, frequencies, and atoms of that Presence wherever God inspires you to direct your Presence. I know this sounds a bit "woo-woo" but when you practice using your breath to ground yourself in Presence, you'll find yourself able to - even in stressful, hectic, rushed, busy and crowded scenarios - give your attention to whatever or whoever most needs it. It actually works to visualize a breastplate of Presence and then to charge it with an inhale and send it forward into the world on an exhale.

The world so desperately needs Presence, doesn't it?

In an age of constant distraction, and doing, doing, doing as though we are human doings instead of human beings, most people's Presence is constantly non-existent or shattered. Yet not many authors, preachers or gurus speak of the crucial importance of Presence. Mindfulness, yes. Focus, yes. Awareness, yes. But Presence has an altogether different ring to it when the word is said aloud or envisioned as a breastplate upon one's body.

By definition, *Presence* is a state or fact of existing, occurring, or being present in a place or thing, while being present means becoming fully focused on or involved in what one is doing or experiencing.

I want to help teach that kind of Presence to people. Since that meditation last year, God has placed this upon my heart. I firmly believe that family is foundation, and that before one ventures out into the world to slay dragons or affect change, one must first go to battle for or implement habits and routines in one's own immediate family. So I began by teaching my twin boys River and Terran Presence. Presence with each tiny particle of air in their young inhales and exhales. Presence with each padded footstep sound out of their bed in the morning. Presence with each ray of sunshine that strikes their skin. Presence with every drop of rain that settles on their head during a drizzle. Presence with every bite of food slowly lifted to the lips and savored and chewed. Presence with every sip of wine and olive oil and yes, even water. And of course, Presence, eye contact, care and love for every human with which they interact. Pure, unadulterated Presence must saturate the life of one who wants to be fully connected to loving others and loving God..

How is that Presence broken?

Sure, as I've already mentioned, our daily distractions—particularly technology, work, and endless to-do lists—threaten each moment to break our Presence, but I think the vicious cycle of loss of Presence begins when we are young. Think back to your childhood, which is something so many of us fail to regularly do. Remember who you were as a child before you began to feel the pressure to become who you thought the world wanted you to be, rather than the true, authentic self God called you to be. Presence began to fade when it was overwhelmed by all the running, lifting, twisting, twirling, spinning, catching, releasing, starting, ending, consuming, smartphone checking, escaping and endless trying and yearning as you tried to be who the world wanted you to be. As you disconnect from self, that fragile breastplate of Presence remains with you on the constant because you become dissatisfied or disillusioned with the simplicity, contentment and peace of being who God had called you to be.

But if you return to this Presence by learning to pause, breathe and halt your dancing through the bullets of the matrix of life, you once again become connected to your true purpose. You are not ashamed of the purpose statement you will discover in the next chapter, you are not so caught up in the doing that you forget about the being, and you have deep knowing that if you cannot be present, then there is too much.

You know what I mean. Too much to do. Too much to tend to. Too much to make. Too many promises to keep. Too much business to tend to. Emails to write. Books to read. Tests to take. School to do. Podcast to listen to. Phone calls to dial. Rooms and garages to clean. New hobbies and toys to try. Mail to open. Mail to send. Yes, yes, yes to all the shiny pennies and "opportunities" accompanied by a relative lack of "no, this distracts me from Presence." These tasks and to-do lists can all seem very laudable, honorable and productive, but at the end of the day result in little meaningful impact versus focusing with excellence upon one fully present task done well or one fully present conversation that leaves someone feeling truly cared about because you took the time, looked into someone's eyes, listened with patience and loved.

Until that meditation session, until I truly realized what Presence truly was, my purpose statement was "to empower people to live a more joyful, adventurous, and fulfilling life." But I realize now that this purpose statement doesn't place me in the present, and indeed, tempts me to be and even paints me into a corner of being some kind of strong, chest-thumping warlord who leads people on adventure quests in a never-ending cycle of unfulfilling *doing*. I have no regrets about that purpose statement, for it served me well during my days of a cowboy-athlete-jester-entertainer-adventure.

But I have learned, as you will discover within the pages of this book, that it is time to rise to a greater calling as a father, leader and king. So what is my *true* purpose statement after much reflection and introspection upon the importance of Presence?

I'll tell you (and in the next chapter, I'll tell you how I formed this purpose statement, and how you can form your own purpose statement too):

... "To Read & Write, Learn & Teach, Sing & Speak, Compete & Create In Full Presence & Selfless Love, To The Glory Of God."

Summary

I feel a deep sense of Presence as I think of and live out that purpose statement, and if I can go forth and love others with that purpose statement while remaining fully present, then I know deep in my soul that I will be living as God has truly called me to live.

So I now commit, I promise and I prioritize for the rest of my days, to wearing this breastplate of Presence, and to sharing Presence with others in as deep and meaningful a way as I can, from the first breath I take upon waking, to the first step I take when my feet touch the ground out of bed, to the first sip of water that touches my lips and onwards into every experience and interaction of the day.

How about you? Do you plan to be more present? Perhaps you need some accountability in doing so, or even more people in your life upon which to "practice" your presence. So now it's time to connect with friends, old and new.

For resources, references, links and additional reading and listening material for this chapter, visit FitSoulBook.com/Chapter2.

CHAPTER III

DON'T LET OLD FRIENDS DIE

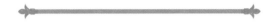

Ever heard of the five regrets of the dying?

Made popular by palliative care practitioner Bronnie Ware's online article *"Regrets of The Dying"* and later transformed into the newly published book *Top Five Regrets of the Dying: A Life Transformed by the Dearly Departing*, these five regrets most often uttered by those on their deathbed are as follows:

- *I wish I'd had the courage to live a life true to myself, not the life others expected of me.*

- *I wish I hadn't worked so hard.*

- *I wish I'd had the courage to express my feelings.*

- *I wish I had stayed in touch with my friends.*

- *I wish that I had let myself be happier.*

While each of these regrets could be addressed in great detail, I'd like you to especially think today about the fourth regret: I wish I had stayed in touch with my friends. Bronnie says:

> *"Often they would not truly realise the full benefits of old friends until their dying weeks and it was not always possible to track them down. Many had become so caught up in their own lives that they had let golden friendships slip by over the years. There were many deep regrets about not giving friendships the time and effort that they deserved. Everyone misses their friends when they are dying.*
>
> *It is common for anyone in a busy lifestyle to let friendships slip. But when you are faced with your approaching death, the physical details of life fall away. People do want to get their financial affairs in order if possible. But it is not money or status that holds the true*

*importance for them. They want to get things in order more for the
benefit of those they love. Usually though, they are too ill and weary
to ever manage this task. It all comes down to love and relationships
in the end. That is all that remains in the final weeks, love and
relationships."*

I recently revisited Bronnie's article and meditated upon how those words apply to my own life.

See, if you ask my parents, they'll both tell you, as they have told me and as I already know about myself, that I never liked to hang out with people too much. I was introverted and had a few very close friends, most often three to four at a time maximum, with whom—aside from my two brothers—I spent the majority of my time.

For the most part, I was never into being popular or hanging out with large crowds, and particularly disliked parties and large gatherings, during which I'd often duck away by myself or with just one to two others for more meaningful and connected time together.

But those few close friends were indeed very dear to me. I remember each of their names: Gerad, Luke, Brian, Matt, Bill, and Grant, namely.

Yet oddly enough, I realized as I was reading about the five regrets of the dying, that it's been years—no, *decades*—since I've spoken so much as a word to these dear old friends.

Life happened.

I moved on.

They moved on.

We started careers and built families and became responsible adult males, sadly with pruned away friendships.

It seemed so easy to let yet another year go by without reaching out or checking in with these old friends, and slowly those old friends began to slip away. I began to forget what they talked like, what they looked like, what they smelled like, and what it felt like to be with them. I forgot their seven digit phone numbers I had memorized back before the days of smartphones, forgot which city they lived in or whether they'd recently moved and forgot how many kids they had and how old those kids were, culminating in a near total disconnect from the very souls I had surrounded myself with all during childhood.

Perhaps you have experienced the same.

If you're a man reading this, then it's very much more likely you have experienced this, as research has shown that men seem to be even less adept than women when it comes to forming new friends or staying in touch with old friends.

Why is this important? Why should you care? Why shouldn't you just let your current suite of co-workers, neighbors, family, and tennis or golf buddies replace all those old friends?

Here are just a few of the reasons I can think of:

• *Old friends remind us who we are at our core.* As you learned in Chapter 8, the kind of things you enjoyed doing and were good at as a child are likely the same kind of things that will help you feed your soul's primary purpose now. There's nothing like reminiscing with old friends, who know exactly who you have been and where you're from, to maintain those memories from childhood and stay connected to who you once were, and likely still are. Memories fade, but what is remembered remains.

• *Old friends tend to more readily accept you for who you are.* The people you grew up with and celebrated childhood with tend to be far more understanding of you and your strengths and weaknesses than brand new folks who you've never met. They remember when you peed your pants on the roller coaster, when you got tipsy for the first time at a party, and when you got four straight F's in math. Sharing those kinds of early mistakes and memories creates a near judgment-free zone that allows you to hang out with old friends without feeling the pressure to be anyone other than who you are.

• *Old friends are fun to be with, even if you don't like to do the same things.* The bonds from childhood go far beyond common interests. They are solid with firm foundations and deep like the roots of an old tree. So when you look up your high school bestie and they're running a vegetable oil-laden fast food chain empire while you're a naturopathic physician or holistic nutritionist, guess what? It seems so much easier to set those differences and strange career opposites aside and simply hang out and be friends again.

• *Old friends allow for enjoyable, nostalgic remembrances.* There's nothing like snorting wine out your nose at dinner and rolling with laughter until your gut hurts as you recall those times your successful executive CEO friend you've reconnected with farted embarrassingly on his first date, the time you pranked your teacher with hot sauce in ketchup, or how you both used to stand in front of the mirror and pop zits at it, perhaps to bug your mother. In truth, these kinds of hilarious nostalgic memories serve to keep you not only connected to your childhood, but keep you young, too.

• *Old friends tend to stick with you through thick and thin.* Sure, you may have forgotten to talk to them for the past ten years, and you may have let deep friendships pass away into what you thought was a complete non-existence, but when you reconnect, you'll find those old friends are ready to jump right back into friendship no matter who you are or what you've been through in life. Once again, there's just something about being children together that allows you to so much more easily connect and re-connect in adulthood, very similar to how you never really forget to ride a bike, even if you haven't touched it for a decade.

Pair a few of the reasons I've thought above with the writings on the hidden epidemic of loneliness **I express in Chapter 6 and it seems that renewing old friendships could be a very good idea indeed.**

It's Not Good To Be Alone

The Bible—the single book I rely upon most for deep wisdom and insight—has some wonderful examples of the importance of friendships too, beginning with Genesis 2, which reads: "The Lord God said, "It is not good for the man to be alone."

Ecclesiastes 4:9-12 says, *"Two are better than one, because they have a good reward for their toil. For if they fall, one will lift up his fellow. But woe to him who is alone when he falls and has not another to lift him up! Again, if two lie together, they keep warm, but how can one keep warm alone? And though a man might prevail against one who is alone, two will withstand him—a threefold cord is not quickly broken."*

Proverbs 17:17: *"A friend loves at all times, and a brother is born for adversity."*

Proverbs 27:17: *"Iron sharpens iron, and one man sharpens another."*

Then, quite powerfully, there's John 15:13, which says: *"Greater love has no one than this, that someone lay down his life for his friends."*

As I made an effort to reconnect with old friends over the past few weeks, I thought about not only the passages above, but also the following examples of firm and fine friendships in the Bible:

The story of David and Jonathan in 1 Samuel is an inspirational tale of two warrior-brothers who shared a close emotional bond of deep loyalty. 1 Samuel 18 describes their relationship: *"As soon as he had finished speaking to Saul, the soul of Jonathan was knit to the soul of David, and Jonathan loved him as his own soul."*

We can see in this solid friendship a staggering amount of love, loyalty, and emotional openness, which are not surprisingly three traits that modern psychologists have deemed necessary for friendships to thrive.

Then there's Moses and Aaron, two friends who worked together to accomplish great things to the glory of God. See, Moses had a great fear of public speaking. So God appointed Moses' brother, Aaron, as his speaker - and together they accomplished one of the most glorious rescues in all of history: the mass exodus of the Israelites from Egypt—proving what two friends with close bonds can accomplish when they complement each other's strengths and weaknesses.

Elijah and Elisha were prophets of Israel so close to each other that when Elijah declared he was departing to another city, Elisha spoke up and said: *"As the Lord lives, and as you yourself live, I will not leave you."* Elijah was a mentor to Elisha, but he was not only a mentor, he was a friend so close that Elisha swore to God they would never be separated. It didn't matter that Elijah was perhaps older, more intimidating, or more experienced. Age and status become so much less important when someone is your true friend.

Fret not ladies: the friendships in the Bible are not only about men. For example, there's the story of Naomi and her daughter-in-law Ruth. Ruth was married to one of Naomi's sons, and even when Naomi fell on tough times, Ruth pledged her life to the stricken and poor Naomi in Ruth 1:16-17, when she says: "Don't urge me to leave you or turn back from you. Where you go I will go, and where you stay I will stay."

Once again, you can see that friends don't leave friends alone and that no matter how many trials there are to overcome in a friendship, unconditional love and self-sacrifice are common characteristics in lasting, solid friendships.

Finally, the ultimate example of friendship is something that you perhaps discovered when explained to you the ultimate Hero's Journey in Chapter 9—the friendship between us lowly humans and the great king Christ Jesus. Remember John 15:13, quoted above?

"Greater love has no one than this, that someone lay down his life for his friends."

Guess who said that?

If you guessed "Jesus," then you are correct.

We see this statement reflected perfectly in the eventual sacrifice of Jesus, who laid down His valuable and holy life, with absolutely no need to do so, in a demonstration of pure love and sacrifice to us. While I certainly know deep in my soul that our relationship with Jesus goes far beyond friendship, and that he is in fact not just a special friend, but also a king to worship and honor, he would not have uttered this statement had he not considered us to be his dear friends—friends who he was prophesying that he loved so much he would eventually die for.

How To Reconnect

So, based on all this, what did I do to reconnect to old friends?

It was quite simple, really. *It was actually as simple to reconnect to all those old friends as it was to grow distant from them in the first place.*

While social media platforms like Facebook and LinkedIn and search engines like Google and TruthFinder—all of which seem to be able to find just about anyone on the planet with a few swift taps of the finger—certainly have their failings and downsides, the convenient thing about them is that within just a couple minutes, you can usually hunt down most or all of those old friends and easily contact them.

And that's what I did.

"Hey Gerad, long-time, no-see man! How's the family?"

"Brian, dude, I was randomly thinking of you the other day. How's life, man?"

"Bill - holy cow! It's been years and I had a dream the other night about us playing video games in your basement. What are you up to these days?"

You get the idea.

The result was quite meaningful and satisfactory. I called one friend and chatted for an hour, and another for twenty minutes. I met one at a coffee shop and shared a cup of coffee while we reminisced on old times. I visited another at his place of work and surprised him with an awkward handshake, then a firm, long-neglected hug.

I learned of marriages and divorces, new children and children starting college, prayer requests and needs, interesting hobbies and novel careers I never would've expected from that old friend, and much more. Each encounter resulted in a deep, satisfied smile on my face and smile in my soul that I'd reconnected with not just a human that I'd grown up with, but with a soul that will go on to live forever—a soul too precious to simply walk away from.

The entire process of reconnecting to old friends, was, in a word, amazing; and I now have a Google doc open on a tab in my browser with an ever-expanding list of local new friends who I can invite to dinner parties, backyard barbecues, frisbee golf, or the tennis court—along with a list of old, once-forsaken friends who I can occasionally hit up on Facebook messenger, my phone, or in-person when I happen to be near their city.

How about you? After reading this, do you plan on connecting to at least one old friend? How about maintaining that list of old friends, and adding in all your new friends, too, so that anytime you have a free evening or open weekend, you can step out, make phone calls, send out invitations, arrange meet-ups, and foster relationships?

I would encourage you—no, challenge you—to do so, and to not delay. Do it today. Do it now. All it takes is a text, a Facebook message, or even scrolling through your ancient phone contacts to find that one number you haven't dialed in so many years, and a simple message such as "Hey INSERTNAMEHERE, it's been a really long time. I randomly thought of you today. How's life?" Go ahead, do it. If you find or have found yourself frustrated that friends and relationships still seem to easily fade away, even after re-sparking connections, or that you still have difficulty building new relationships with acquaintances or co-workers, then you'll definitely want to tune into the next chapter.

For resources, references, links and additional reading and listening material for this chapter, visit FitSoulBook.com/Chapter3.

CHAPTER IV

TIME & TRUST

I have been known to be short, harsh and abrupt when I write emails and texts, interact with people on channels such as Slack and Asana, and even talk to folks on social media platforms like Facebook and Instagram.

A typical digital interaction with me often goes something like this:

Email from fan: *"Hey Ben, I hope your day is going fantastically! I really loved how you laid out your entire recipe for that killer salad, then followed it up with the how-to smoothie video. You really inspire me, man. I have a huge favor/question to ask of you: can you let me know what your favorite book is for learning about healthy food preparation? Thank you so much!"*

My email reply: *"Yeah, search for 'healthy food book' on my website."*

No compliment sandwich.

No winky face or other feel-good emoticon.

No gracious gushing thanks.

Just a strict, short, stoic, Spartan-esque business response. Efficiency at all costs, right?

Or this Slack message, coming from me to a social media employee: *"You spelled workout wrong. It is 'work out.' Pls fix."*

Or this Voxer message, coming from me to a virtual assistant: *"Find me organic coconut flakes by Monday, thx."*

Or this reply to an email from a physician telling me about how excited she was about her cool new stem cell video series, via two highly descriptive paragraphs that finished with asking me whether I wanted to check out a preview of the videos. My curt response? *"Not for now."* (Admittedly, that last one was one of those convenient

Gmail smart composes, which can often aggravate this problem, although it tends to be slightly more polite than me.)

You've probably experienced the same thing.

Digital interactions make it incredibly easy to treat people like computers—simply a series of 0s and 1s that we say random things to in order to make other things happen. It's even worse if you're running a company digitally, like I do.

Why?

As a "virtual" CEO and founder of my nutrition supplements company, Kion, I rarely see my employees, or give them high-fives, or hug them, or look them in the eye, or ask them how their day went, or see if they want to go hit some tennis balls that evening because they are, well, largely *digital to me in nearly all our interactions.* As a result, they can simply be perceived by me as tiny, virtual "coin-bots." I deposit X number of dollars into their bank account each month, and in return, they make Y things happen that results in Z outcomes for the business. What an efficient, logical, well-organized, tidy little factory!

Here are your marching orders and a coin. A hat and two cymbals. Now dance, monkey, dance.

And if things go wrong, or I am delivered results that are anything but perfect? I tend to be baffled. After all, it should be so simple, right? I say X, you do Y, and Z happens. If anything goes wrong in that logical chain of events, then you're an idiot, because it's all spelled out and you're supposed to be able to do your task *just like a computer*, darn-it. After all, you kind of are a computer to me since I'm always talking to you through one. Or a machinery-driven monkey, if you'd like to think of it that way.

The same transactional scenario can happen with customers and clients, especially those with whom I interact with online. They can simply be tiny, virtual "coin-bots." They pay me X dollars per month for Y services, such as a diet plan, fitness plan, 20-minute phone call, etc., etc., etc., and I then deliver those services to them, and the business is done, with near-zero consideration given to getting to know them on a more deep, personal level; understand their fears, worries, hopes, or dreams; know the names of their wife or children, or actually recognize them as real people. They are instead texts and font shapes, sound waves traveling through a phone or app, and pixelated, digital avatars who I cannot sense, touch, feel, smell, or fully appreciate in all their beautiful humanness.

Worse yet, once these kinds of impersonal digital interactions become a habit in your life (as they have very much become in mine), *real face-to-face interactions seem to transform into a similar scenario.*

That grocery store clerk ringing up my groceries? Nod, hand over the credit card, take groceries, leave. She's the human "computer" ringing up my sparkling water and macadamia nuts. Who cares about her actual life or how her day is going? That would not be efficient, timely, or machine-like, which is what I've been trained to do in my virtual interactions.

The sweet, lovely gal who takes care of my printing and shipping needs, collects packages and mail from the mailbox, drives my kids to tennis and jiu jitsu, and runs errands for me? Quite similar to the way in which I might send an employee a quickly written and emotionless text or email task, I'll call to her as I'm down working at the kitchen table: *"Get the mail by one. Thanks."* That's it. Nothing about how her day is going or how she slept or if she's feeling well or what exciting things she may have done over the weekend. No real, meaningful connection. Just business as usual, often in a reactive, frantic, and machine-like fashion.

In these scenarios, no longer are real, flesh-and-blood people, actual people. No longer are they precious, unique spirits and souls who you may live with for eternity and beyond. No longer are they understandably flawed in a creative and magically imperfect way, but they are instead a walking flesh-and-blood computer with a chip that sometimes malfunctions and doesn't do or say what you had desired or anticipated, easily treated as a commodity rather than as a fellow human being. People are reduced to tiny cymbal-donning monkeys, there to entertain your economic impulses.

There's actually a name for this increasingly common phenomenon: *transactional relationships.*

WHAT IS A TRANSACTIONAL RELATIONSHIP?

Look, I don't know who coined the term transactional relationship, but I first learned about it from my friend Benjamin Hardy, who details transactional relationships quite elegantly in his Medium article *"How to Create Rare And Life-Changing Relationships With Anyone (even your heroes)."*

Hardy describes transactional relationships as largely economic, functional, and based on an exchange of money, goods, or services. These types of transactional relationships serve a very clear point, and when that point no longer makes sense or has been fulfilled, the transactional relationship ends. You buy your groceries from a grocer, your home from a real estate agent, your suit from a tailor, then perhaps wave goodbye and never see them again or engage in any future meaningful interactions with them.

By their very nature, transactional relationships are about getting the most you possibly can in exchange for as little as possible on your part. They're all about you, and what you can get. Not about what you can give or the deep, important connections that can potentially result from an interaction with a fellow human.

One way to determine whether you treat relationships as transactional is to ask yourself: Do you view "your people" as objects or as people? If the answer is the former, then the relationship is a transaction and merely a means to an end. In such a transactional relationship, there is no intimacy, and instead, everything is pure business. The relationship becomes an item and the meaning becomes a transaction.

If there was a true relationship, the person who is part of the interaction with you might feel an element of love, of trust, and of caring or kindness. They might feel protected. When that person, let's say one of your employees or co-workers, feels protected, they're willing to be more transparent with you, more willing to share what's on their mind, more human, and even able to be more proactive, creative, and productive because they're willing to take risks that may result in failure. Sure, a failure might be something that still needs to be addressed and fixed, but that failure doesn't matter as much on a deep, personal level because your relationship with them goes beyond a pass-fail, black-and-white, transactional relationship, and is instead of understanding and accepting of them as a fellow human being. The relationship goes beyond a mere transaction. The hairstylist who messed up your bangs isn't someone you crucify with a nasty Google review and who is going to be scared for her next dozen hair appointments because of how you've treated her but is instead willing to move on and rise to the occasion because you laughed with her, hugged it out, and talked with her about how she was distracted because her kid is at home with the stomach flu. Get it?

In contrast, Hardy describes in his article how, if a person doesn't feel protected in a relationship, they won't speak up. They won't share what's on their mind or take risks. Instead, they pander to the relationship, don't act in their power, and act like a victim. This is because transactional relationships won't protect a person. If they don't show up how they're supposed to show up, they're not protected. Instead, they're rejected.

I've personally seen this happen in many of my relationships. A book editor who is afraid to proactively point out to me potential chapter improvements in my book because of my tendency to comment robotically and rudely on her proposed fixes with mere "Yes, do this." or "No, don't do that."

A personal assistant who won't approach me about something I do that bothers or offends them because we don't have a deep personal relationship, but instead a "show up, get paid, do your job, go home" transactional relationship. So they silently put their head down, work, and go home—still offended.

A child who isn't creative and free-flowing on a book report due to my tendency to red pen an essay, hand it back, and give them their deadline to fix, without chatting with them about how the book made them feel on a deep emotional level or even how their day is going.

As I've learned more about the nature of transactional relationships and my propensity to engage in them, I began to ask myself: When did I start thinking of people as "transactions" instead of deep, human souls?

How I Became Transactional

I grew up observing my grandfather and my father's serial entrepreneurship and, at quite a young age, became quite the little entrepreneur myself.

For example, as a young boy, I would save all my Halloween candy under my bed, then—when summer rolled around and king-sized Butterfingers, Halloween colored Nerds candy, and other fringe novelty sugar items were scarce—I would sell it to the other neighborhood kids and families in our homeschooling co-op.

As a teenager, I ran a successful neighborhood babysitting business and tennis coaching business, which is how I saved up much of my college money and how I also continued to realize that people have the potential to be not just people—but also "opportunities to build a business."

Throughout college, I painted homes, hustled for tips while working at a pub and coffee shop, traveled through the city doing private in-residence, high-end personal training, made croissants and cappuccinos at a French bakery early in the morning, and engaged in all manner of enterprises that surely helped solidify within me a respectable work ethic and knowledge of business, but that no doubt continued to foster my tendency towards seeing people as a means to an end. Other human beings could help me fulfill the base of Maslow's hierarchy of needs, pay the bills, and chock away a few coins in the hat for a rainy day.

But then things got even worse.

After graduating from college and managing my gyms and personal training studios for half a decade, I launched an online business. People not only continued to become transactions but also digital 0s and 1s who I didn't even have to physically be with. I could hide behind a screen and bark orders. I could be faceless and emotionless, operating from a mentality of pure and strict business via a few taps of the keyboard to communicate with anyone, anywhere in the world. Eventually, there were no more Friday night parties with personal training clients, lunchtime forays with co-workers, hugs with customers who needed a little love, daily eye-to-eye interactions, high-fives, handshakes, or anything else that might have allowed for transactional relationships to become transformational. Lack of need for empathy and emotion can become so easily built into largely online and digital relationships, and this phenomenon certainly became woven into my life.

Digital clients.

An online company.

Working remotely.

Communicating primarily with virtual assistants or via computers, phones, software, and apps.

Is being a serial entrepreneur and having the ability to run entire companies via the internet a convenience? Yes.

Is it also able to transform one into an impersonal, fully transactional asshole who views work as a transactional process void of emotion? Also, sadly, yes. Ironically, even when able to engage in transformational relationships with people such as my wife, my children, or my close friends, the majority of my relationships that had anything to do with business became almost purely transactional. That was just my very flawed impression of how the world works.

Why You Too Can Easily Slide Into A Transactional Relationship Mentality

Let's face it: Transactional relationships existed long before society's evolution into digital work.

From the horrors of slavery to the mistreatment of factory workers during the industrial revolution to unfair wages historically paid to women and children, one can find examples of the travesty of transactions throughout history.

So what is the reason that relationships can become transactional?

Sure, I think a lack of love and truly caring for our fellow human beings can be part of the problem.

Certainly so can selfishness, greed, ungratefulness, or any other sinful and self-seeking character tendency.

But in my opinion, especially because I've seen many people, including myself—who actually do deeply care for others and love others, and who do via family and friendships display that they can create transformational relationships—nonetheless fall into the transactional relationship trap...

...the tendency to engage in transactional relationships comes down to navigating through life in a hurry, with an attitude of scarcity, of time and resources, and a particular perception that there just isn't enough time in the day to treat every human in every interaction in a way that a human being should be treated and honored.

There's not enough time to write a few extra lines in an email showing that you actually care.

Not enough time to pick up the phone and call instead of sending an emotionless text.

Not enough time to chat with the grocery store clerk about how his or her day is going because, after all, you're late for an appointment.

Not enough time to hug someone, look someone in the eye, or pause to engage in human connection because you're rushing to your next important task.

That's right: If you navigate through life with a belief in the scarcity of time, it's going to be very, very easy for you to engage in rushed and shallow transactional relationships that leave people feeling as though they're simply a stepping stone to your next checkbox in life.

HOW TO GIVE YOURSELF THE TIME TO TRULY TREAT PEOPLE AS PEOPLE

So what's the opposite of scarcity of time?

Trust.

The single biggest obstacle to you feeling as though there actually will be enough time to show people that you care, to ask people questions and engage in conversations blanketed in kindness and love, to be fully present in your interactions with others, and to provide a space of empathy, of listening and of connection is an absence of trust.

See, to be overwhelmed with a sense of peace that there will be enough time in the day to accomplish everything you need to accomplish and still have time left over for treating people the way they deserve, you must operate with a spirit of an abundance of time and a trust that God will provide, even if you are ten minutes late for a post-lunch appointment because you took the time at lunch to chat about life with a co-worker or employee.

Trust that God will care for you. Trust that the time will be there. Trust that abundance will outpace scarcity.

But if you *lose trust* and you suddenly *thrust time to the top of the totem pole of priorities*, then eventually time comes before people, and people become transactional.

So your choice in terms of which direction your relationships go looks something like this:

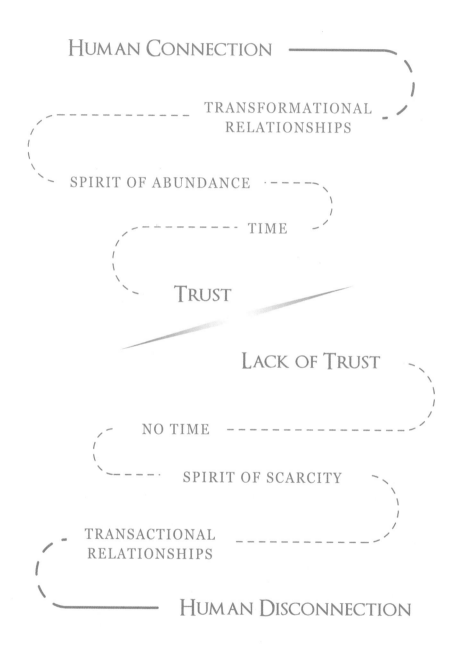

HUMAN CONNECTION

TRANSFORMATIONAL RELATIONSHIPS

SPIRIT OF ABUNDANCE

TIME

TRUST

LACK OF TRUST

NO TIME

SPIRIT OF SCARCITY

TRANSACTIONAL RELATIONSHIPS

HUMAN DISCONNECTION

Make sense?

If it does, then simply take a second this week to ask your restaurant waiter how their day is going.

Pause, and take one minute to write a couple of extra lines in that email you'd normally hurry through and send off without emotion.

Try to create just one comment to the house cleaner or plumber or landscaper or anyone else who you normally find yourself tempted to treat coldly and in a business-like fashion. Ask them about how their weekend was, or how their kids are, or what they're doing for fun that night.

Just start small.

It takes less time than you'd think to make a human connection. You just have to trust that God will provide and that the time will be there even if you're taking extra minutes out of your day to connect with people meaningfully.

As a matter of fact, the Bible tells us quite clearly why we don't need to operate from a spirit of scarcity. Matthew 6:25-34 says:

> *"Therefore I tell you, do not worry about your life, what you will eat or drink; or about your body, what you will wear. Is not life more than food, and the body more than clothes? Look at the birds of the air; they do not sow or reap or store away in barns, and yet your heavenly Father feeds them. Are you not much more valuable than they are? Can any one of you by worrying add a single hour to your life?*

> *"And why do you worry about clothes? See how the flowers of the field grow. They do not labor or spin. Yet I tell you that not even Solomon in all his splendor was dressed like one of these. If that is how God clothes the grass of the field, which is here today and tomorrow is thrown into the fire, will he not much more clothe you— you of little faith? So do not worry, saying, 'What shall we eat?' or 'What shall we drink?' or 'What shall we wear?' For the pagans run after all these things, and your heavenly Father knows that you need them. But seek first His kingdom and His righteousness, and all these things will be given to you as well. Therefore do not worry about tomorrow, for tomorrow will worry about itself. Each day has*

enough trouble of its own."

That's right: Each day has enough trouble of its own.

So be nice.

Don't be a monster to people.

Don't be the ultra-successful go-getter who doesn't have anybody show up at their funeral because they were an asshole.

Care, and don't just say you care, show you care. Take the time. You're not going to starve or miss a house payment or lose all your fitness gains or not finish a work deadline because you took the time to care for a fellow human being. If anything, you're going to be a happier, more peaceful person—and they will be too.

A FEW OTHER TIPS TO CREATE TRANSFORMATIONAL RELATIONSHIPS

In addition to trusting and having a spirit of abundance instead of scarcity, you may want to consider a few of the tips that are detailed in two helpful pieces of content that I'll link to on the resources page for this chapter: Laura Mazzullo's *"Transactional: is that REALLY who you want to be?"* and Benjamin Hardy's *"How to Create Rare And Life-Changing Relationships With Anyone (even your heroes),"* including:

Assume the best intentions in others. Ask yourself: "What would happen if I assumed everyone was doing their best?". People usually don't slack, mess up, and commit all-too-common human errors on purpose or out of spite. Most folks, including your family and co-workers, actually do care. But they are fallible humans and not flawless automatons, which is why they have actual personalities, humor, proactiveness, and creativity. So cut them some friggin' slack already.

Be kind. Just. Be. A. Nice. Person. That's all. Care. Smile. Love your fellow human. Say *"thank you"* and *"please"* more often, and not *"thx"* and *"pls."* Heck, even toss in a bit of *"I love you."* or *"I'm grateful for you."* Kindness tends to be kind of contagious actually and makes your day better too.

Provide advice and support, not just correction. Did your marketing manager butcher an email headline or print a brochure with some glaring typos. Sure...point it out, but perhaps ask how you could help them avoid such understandable errors in the future (*"Can I find someone to help proofread for you?"* or *"Can I purchase you access to Grammarly or give you some tips on how to use it?"*)—all in kindness and assuming the best intention on their part, of course.

Imagine your digital interactions are physical. Write your emails the same way you'd say something to someone's face (*"Yo."* can become *"Hey, how's your day going man?"*). Send a text as though you were looking into someone's eyes (*"Umm...OK."* can become *"Can you explain a little bit more what you mean by that, I don't quite understand?"*). Introduce colleagues or make connections as though you were seated at dinner together (*"John meet Ben, Ben meet John."* can become *"John, you have to meet Ben. You guys are such kindred spirits, I know it. You guys have to hang out sometime, or at least get on the phone together for a bit."*). The feel of real physical connection can still happen when connecting in our digital era. And yes, I know it takes more time. That's where trust fits in, remember?

Don't see people as dollar signs. See people as people. Sure, they may be a paying customer, a producing employee, or a potential client, but the fact that we often exchange goods or services in exchange for other goods and services with these type of folks doesn't mean that at the end of the day they're also not a mother, a father, a brother, a sister, a parent, a person who loves tennis or the outdoors or cooking, and someone with just as many faults, flaws, worries, joys, F-ups, addictions, weird habits, and unorganized desks as you. We're all messy humans and we all need stuff from each other. Let's just not make needing stuff the ultimate objective of our interactions, OK? Let's instead make the ultimate objective love and connection.

Be transformational. Finally, Ben Hardy, in the same article I mentioned earlier, describes the opposite of a transactional relationship. He calls it a transformational relationship. Transformational relationships can start out as transactions. But they then go far beyond the mere exchange of money, goods, or services—and are instead about giving the most you possibly to help others and advance others' in a synergistic and win-win way. In transformational relationships, you have lots of protection, which is important because as I alluded to earlier, feeling protected is the key to doing invaluable work, which you just can't do without the love, help, and support of others. For example, Ben describes how he hired someone named Joel to help him with his communication skills. But that relationship stopped being transactional very quickly. They connected deeply. They started serving and helping each other. And

Joel has helped Ben in ways he could never help himself. In fact, Ben says Joel changed his life. He goes on to say:

> *"Your relationship isn't transformational if it doesn't change you. If you're not getting better. And if there aren't generous gifts given without compulsion. Your relationship isn't transformational if it's primarily about you. Your relationship isn't transformational if you're not creating a bigger pie — both for the relationship and all involved. But beyond that, your relationship isn't transformational if you aren't making the world a better place. Your relationships aren't feeling protected is the key to doing invaluable work. Because you can't do your best work without the love, help, and support of others. if you don't truly love the people you're with. If you aren't genuine. If you're not thoughtful."*

Once you recognize and identify the relationships and interactions in your life that have become transactional, the steps above become clear and easy to take. It's just a matter of knowing the seriousness of the matter, then taking action. I trust that you're now equipped to do just that.

Summary

So, world, I'm sorry.

I'm sorry I've been an asshole.

I'm sorry I've been transactional.

I'm sorry I've treated you like a digital 0 and 1, a pixelated avatar, and a coin-bot computer.

I'm ready for my relationships to become transformative. Life is too short and people are too magical for it to be any other way.

Please forgive me.

How about you? Have you slid, like I have, into largely transactional relationships with people, even those who you love and interact with on a daily basis? Will you join me in, instead, committing to transformational relationships?

Then I challenge you to start here: Take one relationship that is currently a transactional relationship for you, and take a truly transformative, caring step towards making the transactional transformational. How about a phone call to an employee instead of a text? A "how is your day going?" to the grocery store clerk instead of a curt nod and half-smile? An email that, despite still being efficient, actually shows that you're human and they're human, such an "I'm so grateful for you today" in your salutatory greeting? You get the idea. Speaking of relationships, there is, in my opinion, no more important relationship than that which you form with those tiny, impressionable humans who you may interact with on a daily basis in your own household. So whether you have children, plan to have children or hang out regularly with children, the next chapter is for you.

For resources, references, links and additional reading and listening material for this chapter, visit *FitSoulBook.com/Chapter4.*

CHAPTER V

MAKE EVERY MOMENT COUNT?

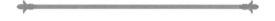

Three weeks ago, someone commented to me that I ought to "make every moment count" with my kids, because 99% of the time parents spend with their children occurs before those children are eighteen years old, after which our precious offspring are theoretically out of the house, out and about living their own adventures, starting their own families, and largely inaccessible for the rest of a parent's lifetime to be available to spend quality time with that parent.

After being told this, in addition to me quickly recalling the fact that 87% of statistics are made up on the spot (heh), I found myself reminiscing on a verse from Harry Chapin's *"Cat's In The Cradle"* song...

> *"...when you comin' home son?... I don't know when...but we'll get together then Dad...you know we'll have a good time then...".*

Furthermore, I found myself calling bullsh*t on this entire "scarcity-of-time" with kids concept.

I mean, *really?*

We *really* need to feel the pressure that 99% of the hours we'll ever spend with our children will have been spent with them by the time they're eighteen years old? Really?

I'll tell you one thing I know for a fact: If that skewed time curve of quality time occurs between generations of Greenfields, and if my twin boys simply pop in every once in a while to say hello, for a total of 1% of the time I'll ever spend with them after they're eighteen years old, then I would highly suspect something had gone terribly wrong with the Greenfield family model.

THE PROBLEM WITH
"MAKING EVERY MOMENT COUNT"

You're no doubt familiar with the concept that to truly make your life meaningful and impactful, you should live each day as if it was your last. Future thinking. Deathbed thinking. Write your own obituary thinking. Make every moment count, and I-mean-every-last-one-darn-it thinking. You know what I'm talking about.

Walk to your mailbox as though it were your final stroll to retrieve a package.

Go hit the gym as though it was the concluding moment of your life and the last chance with which you'll ever be blessed to move your body.

Have a family dinner as though it were the very last supper of your lives together.

Live your entire life as though your deathbed waiteth, just around the corner.

Now don't get me wrong, we should not—as John Piper so eloquently teaches in his book *Don't Waste Your Life*—waste our lives. We should not spend the day neglecting our life's purpose and instead whittling away at sticks, drawing paintings in the mud with our toes, and staring at the clouds—all while waiting for the next night of sleep to arrive before rinsing, washing, and repeating in a kind-of productive Groundhog Day scenario. That's, of course, the polar opposite of living as though each day were your last.

But neither should we feel the intense magnitude of pressure that arises from a constancy of death-bed thinking.

That walk to the mailbox? Maybe you need to check the weather on your phone while walking, it's not the time to breathe in every last rose petal particle that wafts into your nose as you pause slack-jawed to watch a beautiful butterfly, and you instead need to be back in the kitchen in two minutes to help your spouse clean the dishes.

That trip to the gym? Maybe you don't need to act as though you'll never get a chance to sweat or lift heavy things again, you feel no urge to shout a Braveheart-esque "FREEDOM!" at the top of your lungs as you bench press the heaviest weight of your life, and maybe you simply desire to crank out a few push-ups and intervals on the rowing machine before you jet back to the office. Sure, you can be fully *present and mindful* during that time at the gym, but there's a difference between presence, mindfulness, and the creation of every second spent exercising into an epic battle movie.

And that family dinner? Well, that brings me to perhaps the most important point and the main thrust of this chapter: perhaps you don't need to spend every family dinner solemnly discussing the family trust, legacy, and constitution, while raising eloquent toasts to your children with the finest of wines and engaging in an Epicurean feast of masterful cookery and magnificent proportion because...who knows? You gotta make every moment count, right? This could very well be your last dinner, after which you will crawl up to bed, wiping chicken skin and gravy juices off your face, and pass quietly away of a heart attack in your sleep at 1 AM.

No doubt the issue with this kind of thinking is as clear to you as it seems to me: It threatens to make life just a bit too dreary, a bit too dark, a bit too dramatic, and a bit too skewed towards a stressful scenario in which every moment must not only count, but also be so absolutely epic that you have no clue how you'll top it in the next moment—but perhaps it can include purchasing a new Harley-Davidson to motor out to the mailbox, finally having the courage to wear that yellowish cheetah-themed leotard suit to the gym, and celebrating the next family dinner with the governor, on a spaceship, wearing top hats.

What Is Better Than Making Every Moment Count?

So if you shouldn't shirk your duties in the joy derived from fully engaging in your life's purpose, including being with your children, and you also shouldn't feel the pressure to transform every last second into an epic movie moment—how should you approach this concept of "spending quality time" with loved ones (because, after all, as we've established from somewhat sketchy statistics, you just never know how long they'll be around)?

I'll tell you the answer, and it's quite simple: don't feel the pressure to make every moment count. But do try to make every moment *memorable*.

That's right: *make every moment memorable.*

Here's what I mean...

...your children will appreciate and get just as much value out of building their new Lego kit with you on the patio for an hour every Saturday as they will a random summer weekend afternoon based upon a jam-packed itinerary that includes a trip to the zoo, ice cream cones, the arcade, and a movie, culminating with a sleepover in the backyard tree fort.

...they also care more about gathering as a family to sing the doxology before each dinner and eat Dad's famous eggs and waffles breakfast-for-dinner for the weekly Tuesday night feast than they do a trip to a fancy steakhouse for which you mortgaged your car so they could each order a bone-in ribeye...

...they aren't going to value a tricked-out Tesla road trip to the coast as much as they value you singing at the top of your lungs every single time your favorite oldies tune comes on the radio when you drive them to the park to play on Wednesday afternoons...

...they'd rather go on the monthly family hike to a camp spot 20 miles from your house than they would hop on a last-minute flight deal to Cabo to live at a fancy resort far from home for five days...

...they'd rather play the thrice-weekly game of cards (ours are Exploding Kittens, Unstable Unicorns, and, my favorite Bears vs. Babies) at the dinner table, than they would help you plan out your final will or testament or have a serious family-planning meeting about bank accounts, corporate structure and your grand vision for their future...

...and they'll remember far more fondly that tiny chocolate they always got to munch on every year, each morning, during the 24 day Advent calendar leading up to Christmas day than the fancy iTouch wrapped in gold-flecked wrapping paper under the tree.

Do you spot the distinct difference between the "memory" examples I just gave you? The fancy, expensive, epic moments certainly count but the simple, reliable, fully present, and traditional moments are more memorable.

I'll say it again: don't feel the pressure to make every moment count. But *do* make every moment *memorable*.

TRADITION MAKES MOMENTS BETTER

The traditions, behaviors and actions your family engages in again and again and the regular rituals that you perform at the same time or in the same way on a dependable basis, will serve as the lifeblood of your family. They are the strong fabric that fortifies the knit canvas of your relationship with your children. They are the rocks upon which families and legacies are built.

Traditions can be big, such as an annual trip to the coast, or small, such as Sunday afternoon family tennis. But each is ideally calendared and designed with forethought, intentionality, and purpose. In *The Book of New Family Traditions,"* author Meg Cox defines these types of traditional rituals as "any activity you purposefully repeat together as a family that includes heightened attentiveness and something extra that lifts it above the ordinary ruts."

The benefits of traditions abound.

They offer children dependency, comfort, and security—such as the card game with Mom and Dad that they can rely upon at the end of a stressful school day or the breakfast date with Dad on Wednesdays to get an Acai bowl and go for a walk. They strengthen family bonds by forcing repeated connection and unity in a unique and special environment—such as a monthly trip to an Escape Room. They bestow a sense of identity—tying families to richer cultural and religious history as traditions become embedded into generation upon generation.

They create fond memories of historical or traditional events that have shaped the family and serve as conversation pieces for future times together as you reminisce upon past family pig roasts, trash-talking Scrabble matches, and song-singing expeditions to the local nursing home. They help your children get through tough times—perhaps when the entire family has been uprooted to a new city or state so Dad could get a job, but yet even in this new place, the family can still have their Wednesday night bike rides around the neighborhood. They instill a strong sense of morals and values, especially when centered on spiritual discipline activities such as family prayer, meditation, Bible reading, journaling, and a nighttime bed song.

They create rhythmic, dependable seasons through a child's life—including seasonal activities such as the Spring garden-planting, the Summer morning paddle-boarding trips, the Fall pumpkin carving festival, and the Winter snowman building on the first day of each December. Perhaps most relevant to the idea of your children "disappearing" as you grow old, traditions cultivate the continued involvement of parents and grandparents into a child's life, since they often involve regular excursions, get-togethers, meals, hobbies, events, and activities that engage an entire family together.

In her book, *Ask the Children,* Ellen Galinsky describes a survey in which she asked children what they thought they would remember most about their childhood. The majority of the children responded by fondly recalling simple, everyday traditions like family dinners, holiday get-togethers, and bedtime stories.

Although I didn't personally see all the survey results, I doubt many of the kids expressed fond memories of *"...how Dad took us on a shopping spree to the mall and gave us each a credit card because he thought he might die the next day..."* or *"...when Mom made us stay home from our best friend's 13th birthday party because she was sad that she wasn't going to get to see us when we got older...".*

So moments can certainly count, but they don't need to be epic. They just need to be memorable. Simplicity is OK. Consistency is a must. Dependency is fantastic. Presence is crucial. Weaving these memories into family tradition is more consequential than you may think.

Create simple, consistent, dependable, present moments based on deep-rooted tradition in your family, and you won't need to worry about not seeing your kids once they've flown the nest.

SUMMARY

So you can think about the fact that statistics and "they" say that your child is going to grow up and move out soon, so you better make every moment count. You can dwell on that, feel a bit sad and depressed about it, and paint yourself into a guilt corner as you constantly try to figure out how to ensure no moment is wasted and every moment is supremely epic...

...or...

...you can create a future where you and your family are frequently together until the day you die, including your children, and your children's children - because you *made it so good that everybody wants to stay. They want to keep coming back—for Easter; and Christmas; and Thanksgiving; and Sunday afternoon tennis; and Tuesday night eggs—because you and your family created traditions. You created reunions. You created communities. You created meaning. You created love. You made it so good that everybody wanted to stay.*

If you build your family upon the firm foundation of tradition, then you won't need to worry at all about old age abandonment, long distance, extended, torturous separation from loved ones, or rarely seeing your kids again after they move out.

Make every moment memorable.

And to finish, a blessing to you and your children, and your children's children from one of my favorite little YouTube channels right now: The Yun Family. **Enjoy.**

What do you think? What are your favorite childhood memories and traditions? What memories and traditions are you instilling in your family now? Now that you've learned the importance of your relationship with yourself, your relationship with old friends, and your relationships with young friends, it's time to turn to an important lesson on how to grow and nourish these relationships for life.

For resources, references, links and additional reading and listening material for this chapter, visit FitSoulBook.com/Chapter5.

CHAPTER VI

THE HIDDEN EPIDEMIC

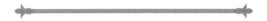

Perhaps it's genetics or perhaps it's because I was homeschooled K-12 in rural Idaho, but I'm an introvert, through and through. Yes, I'm "that guy" at busy conferences who ducks away to my room to go recharge my batteries every few hours - something I can only accomplish by escaping the crowds and being entirely by myself. I thrive on long walks, multi-hour hikes and extended bike rides - usually alone. I become exhausted at networking events and cocktail parties, and often slip away early to sleep, to curl up with a good book, or simply to meditate and breathe. Even at family events, I can often be found off in some quiet corner reading or strumming on my guitar or ukulele.

As a matter of fact, when I was a child, my parents had to coax me, persuade me and yes, even threaten me with punishment, to actually get my nose out of my book and be gracious enough to ever so briefly emerge from my bedroom to say a quick hello to any guests we had at the house, after which I would subsequently rush back to my room and curl up once again with my book (I'd often read until 3 or 4 am and consume several books each day and night!). A multitude of personality tests that I've taken, including the Quiet Revolution test and the Myers-Briggs analysis (both of which I'll link to on the resources page for this chapter), have backed this up: I'm an introvert through and through.

But at the same time, even though I'm completely happy being a loner, I now go out of my way to ensure that (as uncomfortable or unnatural as it was initially for me) I spend plenty of time carving out a couple hours each night for a family dinner and nighttime family rituals, for connecting with old and new friends, for attending networking events, for scheduling plenty of book signings and meet-and-greets, for traveling to crowded conferences, and for actively engaging in local church, community, and charity events. One could even say that I've about halfway transformed myself into a bit of a social butterfly.

So why have I begun to incorporate such a strong emphasis in my life on optimizing friends, charity, community relationships and love - aside from my desire to not be an arrogant, hard-to-approach, uncommunicative a-hole? Turns out, there is a fascinating link between love, family, social connectedness and relationships, and a longer lifespan. This chapter will supply you with a host of practical love tips to include in your own life for a longer lifespan and better health. After all, owning an amazing body and a sharp mind can all be for naught if loneliness, sadness, inflammation, high blood pressure and accelerated aging are all occurring due to lack of friendships, social relationships, community, charity and love - and in this chapter I will teach you exactly why and how to include these important components into your own body, mind and spirit routine.

THE PROBLEM WITH LONELINESS

Imagine a condition that makes a person irritable, depressed, and self-centered, and also increases their risk of dying early by over 25%. Imagine that in industrialized countries, over 30% of folks (a percentage that is increasing at a rapid pace) are afflicted with this condition. Your income doesn't protect you. Nor does your education, your sex, or your ethnicity. Worse yet, the condition is considered to be contagious, damages heart muscle, causes premature death and can affect any ordinary person walking down the street.

This condition exists, and you may already have it. It's called, drumroll please: loneliness. Also known as social isolation, loneliness is often stigmatized, trivialized, and flat-out ignored, but is fast emerging as a worldwide public health problem - oddly enough growing hand-in-hand with so-called "social" media. Worse yet, zero physicians are trained in medical school about how to deal with this problem.

Often, we tend to associate loneliness being homeless, being depressed, being severely introverted or having poor social skills or social anxiety. But none of this is true. Both human and animal longitudinal studies have shown that the deleterious effects of loneliness are not attributable to some fringe subset of isolated individuals, but instead can affect anyone, anywhere.

In addition to the serious emotional toll that you'd expect loneliness to be able to pile upon a human, research has shown that the physical manifestations are also rather grim. Studies have linked loneliness to cancer, cardiovascular disease, inflammation, immune system issues, pain, fatigue, depression, excessive reactivity to stress, rampant elevated cortisol levels and high blood pressure - making the effects of loneliness on part with smoking in terms of mortality risk. Unlike other chronic diseases that tend to wreak havoc more often in aging individuals it's actually young adults who are at the highest risk social isolation.

For example, one recent study found that people who are more lonely show signs of elevated latent herpes virus reactivation and produce more inflammation-related proteins in response to acute stress than did people who felt more socially connected. This suggests that loneliness functions as a chronic stressor that triggers a poorly controlled immune response. During the recent coronavirus pandemic, another series of studies found that participants experiencing interpersonal stressors - including social isolation - had a greater chance of developing upper respiratory illnesses when exposed to cold viruses. Psychological and social stress associated with loneliness were correlated with an overproduction of pro-inflammatory cytokines in response to cold and influenza viruses. This excess of inflammation caused an increased risk of becoming ill. Meanwhile, social integration and social support seemed to offer a protective shield against respiratory infection and illness.

When you think about it, there's a bit of an ancestral context to this whole loneliness problem. Looking at human history from an ancestral standpoint, we see that extended isolation could mean death, since your tribe wasn't physically around to nurture you or protect you. Hence, humans developed social constructs to keep themselves bound together in bands, communities, and tribes, including extended families and social connections that seem to land at around 150 people (that number is actually known today as Dunbar's number).

The frequency and growing epidemic of loneliness is actually a bit ironic, isn't it? Today, we live in a hyper connected society, and yet one of the biggest uphill battles we face in terms of our long-term health is disconnectedness and social isolation. It's far less common than it used to be to know your neighbors by face and name, to engage in face-to-face meet-ups and conversations in connected communities not separated by an electronic barrier, and to be a child raised by an entire tribal community surround you, rather than say, a parent or two, schoolmates you see for a limited amount of time each day, Netflix and a smartphone.

But wait! We walk around with tiny computers in our pockets that can instantly connect us with like-minded peers and people all over the globe. We should be more connected to other people than ever, right? Not quite. Even when you're on Facebook,

Twitter, Snapchat, Instagram, some fringe new platform that's all the rage in Asia and any other social media outlets, you're not actually experiencing relationships the way that you're programmed to and the way that you're hardwired to from an ancestral standpoint. You're not looking into people's eyes, you're not touching them, you're not feeling them and you're not experiencing the invisible, chemical signals that human beings create and ooze from our pores when we're around other human - not to mention the fact that you're missing out on the strong electromagnetic heart and brain signals humans around you constantly emit.

As a matter of fact, a direct relationship between smartphone prevalence and loneliness has started to amass a significant amount of research. For example, a 2015 study showed a correlation between smartphone usage and loneliness in college students. A 2017 study found a significant correlation between attachment anxiety, loneliness, depression and smartphone addiction.

This link between technology and loneliness is even more obvious when you look at smartphone usage in teenagers. An article I recently read in The Atlantic noted that as smartphone usage became more ubiquitous, a rapid and disturbing change in teenage behavior has occurred. These changes began sometime around 2012, when about 50% of Americans owned smartphones (come to think of it, I got my very first iPhone in 2013!). The group born between 1995 and 2012, a group the article dubs "iGen", experienced a significant increase in the use of smartphones and social media. You probably don't fall into that category if you - like me - can't actually remember a time when you actually never even had a smartphone or even really cared about any form of social media at all. In the iGen group, the rates of depression and suicide have significantly increased since 2011. As a matter of fact, teenagers who spend three or more hours per day on electronics have a 35% higher chance of a suicide risk factor and a 27% higher risk of depression. The author of the article notes that "it's not an exaggeration to describe iGen as being on the brink of the worst mental-health crisis in decades. Much of this deterioration can be traced to their phones.".

Each of the social media outlets you use each day make an implicit claim about the structure and organization of human interaction. Instead of direct interaction with others, we are interacting through something metal, something electronic and something impersonal. So the question we should be asking is this: *can we actually form meaningful personal relationships through an impersonal medium?*

Turns out that others have asked (and answered) this same question. Author Sherry Turkle has been studying children's development in technological culture since the late 1970's. In her book *Reclaiming Conversation: The Power of Talk in a Digital Age,* she explains how children use technology, specifically programming, as a form of self-expression. One 13-year old interviewed in the book comments, "When you program a computer, you put a little piece of your mind into the computer's mind and you come to see yourself differently." And you could say that in a way, this self-exploration is personal. It's all about you.

But this kind of personal experience is lacking two things: a relationship, and a prefix. When a significant amount of your time is focused on an impersonal social medium, you miss out on the interpersonal relationships that you can really only get by talking to someone face-to-face. Virtual space has become a place of self-exploration, and dealing with real people, who have a knack for being unpredictable, becomes difficult after spending time in a predictable simulation. Take email for example. In the workplace, it's used to deliberately avoid social interaction, and results in a significant amount of depersonalization. Heck, as you learn in Chapter 4, I'm personally guilty of talking to people more like robots and less like humans when I interact with them virtually. What's worse, when you don't get much interpersonal interaction, your emotional intelligence (EI) - the ability to be able to identify and manage your own emotions and the emotions of others - begins to suffer. People who spend a lot of time on the internet are lonelier, have more "deviant values" (e.g. a willingness to break social norms), and a lack of the robust emotional and social skills characteristic of high EI.

Here's a news flash: when it comes to social isolation and loneliness, it really isn't about getting more friends on Facebook. It isn't about extending your Snapchat streak of chats by yet another week. It isn't about that popup you have set on your computer to reach out via email to some influencer on your digital Rolodex. It isn't about developing the independent, lone-wolf, "I (plus my smartphone) can survive on my own, thank-you-very-much mentality" I personally maintained for so much of my life before I came face-to-face with my own growing loneliness and social isolation. It's about going out of your way to build actual physical, flesh-and-blood relationships and a robust community of people who will come to your rescue when your basement floods, who will show up at your doorstep when you're moving into a new house, and who will cry at your funeral.

Cry at your funeral? Where'd that come from? It's actually a phrase I first discovered in the writings of pastor John Ortberg. Here's what he has to say in his book *I'd Like You More If You Were More Like Me,* which is an essential handbook for developing deep, meaningful, intimate relationships:

"So, who will not be crying at my funeral?

- *my critics*

- *people who write me to ask for favors, but whom I never hear from otherwise*

- *people whose approval I'm constantly trying to gain, but who always withhold it*

- *rich people who I think might give me something if I get to know them better (but so far it hasn't happened)*

- *successful people whose success I think might rub off on me if I hang out with them more often*

- *people who see me frequently but don't remember my name*

- *people who I think could make me feel important if I could just get them to notice me*

- *people who are cooler than I am*

- *famous people I've never actually met*

- *beautiful women whose pictures are on the Internet, but who don't actually know I'm alive*

- *people I'm afraid of*

- *people who are afraid of me*

- *all the people in the little jury box of my mind whose opinion of me matters so much, but who aren't thinking about me at all because they're wondering what other people are thinking about them*

Who is likely to cry at my funeral?

- *my children and their families*

- *my wife*

- *my brother and sister*

- *my good friends*

- *my parents, if I should go before them*

- *people I have genuinely and personally helped*

In other words, the people with whom I have true intimacy.

The question is, Am I giving the best of my time and my life to the people who will cry at my funeral?"

I find it quite interesting that the people who make Ortberg's "cry at my funeral" list aren't really the same people you tend to interact with every day on social media and via email, but rather those people in your life with which you tend to build true, meaningful relationships that keep you from dropping into the dark hole of loneliness. And remember: this is coming from a guy (me) who has 5000 Facebook friends, tens of thousands of Twitter followers, close to half a million Instagram fans, what seems like 8 billion Snapchat messages per day and has still had to deal with intense loneliness.

Anyways, grab Ortberg's book and read it (along with the other books I'll be recommending on the resources page for this chapter) if you want to cut through all the hustle, the hurry, the business and the "I'm too busy to hang out with real, flesh-and-blood people" and to instead develop more meaningful intimacy and relationships in your life. Furthermore, the good news is that you're about to discover how to eliminate loneliness from your life, how to defy social isolation and how to tap into one of the most powerful emotions that exists.

THE OPPOSITE OF LONELINESS: LOVE

In his book *Blue Zones*, longevity expert and author Dan Buettner identified five geographic areas where people live the longest, statistically speaking: Okinawa (Japan), Sardinia (Italy), Nicoya (Costa Rica), Icaria (Greece), and the Seventh-day Adventists in Loma Linda, California.

Buettner offers an explanation, based on empirical data and first-hand observations, as to why these populations live healthier and longer lives. Turns out, the people inhabiting these "blue zones" share common lifestyle characteristics that contribute to their longevity, from life purpose to stress reduction to moderating alcohol intake and beyond. But there are six shared characteristics that are inherent among each and every Blue Zone population. They are:

- *Less smoking*

- *A plant-rich diet*

- *Consistent, moderate physical activity*

- *Consumption of legumes*

- *Family engagement*

And finally...drumroll please:

- *Social interaction*

In his book, Buettner illustrates just how important love is as the unifying factor between family, relationships, social engagement, and community, and even points out the fact that research shows strong social relationships predicts a 50% increased chance of a long, healthy life.

So what is love, exactly? Love actually encompasses a wide variety of emotional and mental states, including the deepest interpersonal affection seen in the intense love between a husband and wife or a mother and child to the simplest pleasure you might experience as you take a delicious bite of cheesecake. The range of definitions of the word love means that the love of a mother differs from the love of a spouse differs from the love of food. Most commonly, love simply refers to a strong feeling of attraction and attachment. Greek philosophers categorized four forms of love: familial love (storge), friendly love (philia), romantic love (eros), and divine love (agape). But love is also an all-encompassing virtue that incorporates kindness, compassion, and affection and perhaps most importantly, an unselfish loyal and benevolent feeling of goodwill towards another.

That's right: having love in your life is not just about the number of your relationships, the strength of your relationships, or how many people love you. Rather, it's the attitude with which you engage in those relationships that predicts a longer and healthier life. While many think that they need to find someone to love them, research shows that the greatest benefits for health, longevity and well-being come not from receiving affection but instead from giving it to others. So perhaps the additional question Ortberg should have posed is: whose funerals will you cry at? As a matter of fact, I tell my children that if they desire true happiness in life, the very greatest thing they can accomplish towards that end is to identify their purpose in life, then to use that purpose to love God and to love others.

Of course, if meaningful love for others and social relationships increases your lifespan, then the opposite must also be true. Drawing on data from four nationally representative longitudinal samples of the U.S. population, one recent study assessed the association of social relationships such as social integration, social support, and social strain with measured biomarkers of physical health like C-reactive protein (an inflammatory marker), systolic and diastolic blood pressure, waist circumference, and body mass index within the life stages of adolescence, young, middle, and late adulthood. The researchers discovered that a higher degree of social integration was associated with lower risk of physiological dysregulation in a dose-response manner, in both early and later life. At the same time, lack of social connections was associated with vastly elevated health risks. Social isolation increased the risk of inflammation by the same magnitude as physical inactivity in adolescence, and the effects of social isolation on hypertension exceeded that of clinical risk factors such as diabetes in old age. This is likely because the same genes impacted by social connection also code for immune function and inflammation. While people with low social connection have higher levels of inflammation, individuals who live a "eudaimonic" lifestyle, defined as a life rich in compassion, altruism (selfless care for others) and a sense of purpose, have surprisingly lower levels of inflammation.

That altruism piece is pretty important too. Take, for example, a study done by Stephanie Brown at the Stony Brook University Medical Center. Those in the study who engaged in helping others and supporting others ended up living longer lives. This was not the case for people who were simply recipients of care and support. Another study supports and extends the findings above, demonstrating that volunteerism predicts a longer life. Interestingly, this second study found that volunteerism lengthened lifespan only when it was performed for purely selfless reasons. When you sincerely wish to help others, you will reap the benefits thereof, so it turns out you cannot deceive your own body about your true intentions for helping others.

This means that while it's important that you're aware that loving others and having lots of love in your life is one of the most potent ways to enhance your wellness and longevity, you shouldn't be going out of your way to experience love so that you can, say, decrease inflammatory cytokines or extend the length of your telomeres. Instead, you should go out of your way to experience love because you actually, genuinely care for your fellow man and fellow woman, because you relish the idea of hanging out with your family and because being with other human beings makes you happy. If you're anything like me, it may take a lot of time, patience and learning to bring yourself to the point where you can shove at the back of your mind the idea that you're attending a family reunion because you care about family and not because you heard it could be good for your physiology, but the more you love others, the more it seems to create a positive cycle in which you love others just because that's what you do not because that's what you should do. Make sense?

Of course, it's tough to love others if you're not actually *around* others. I would know. I used to be the guy at conferences who would stand in the back of the lunchroom with a blank stare on my face, completely paralyzed by the prospect of approaching a table of gabbing attendees to ask for a seat, the student who sat alone in the corner of the university cafeteria with my nose buried in a newspaper, and the fellow who upon first settling into my airplane seat would don my noise-blocking headphones and avoid all eye contact with anyone who seemed to threaten me with an impending conversation.

Then I read a book by author Keith Ferrazzi entitled *Never Eat Alone: And Other Secrets to Success, One Relationship at a Time.* Ferrazzi has a circle of contacts that numbers in the thousands, a circle he's cultivated for years (admittedly, this seems to rub against the concept of Dunbar's number), and a circle that he has built based on what he says is an incredibly important aspect of any relationship: generosity. His approach to never eating alone integrates networking, behavior, intuition, and power, but also emotion, reciprocity, and trust, all integral parts of workplace and personal relationships. Ultimately, I'd sum up his book by saying that it encourages you to find people, sit down at a table with them, and smother them with love by being truly and genuinely interested in them, not striving to "get anything" out of getting to know them, and offering up as much helpful advice as you can give them based on your specific areas of knowledge and expertise. When I walk into a group of people, whether it's a cocktail party, a bar or a conference lunch, this is now my modus operandi. Of course, the book goes into far more detail about how to "never eat alone", and I'd highly recommend you add it to your recommended reading list for this chapter.

Now, it shouldn't be ignored that Ferrazzi's approach actually capitalizes on the connectivity provided by social media and the internet. He described that LinkedIn, Twitter, Facebook and beyond are all powerful tools when used correctly and in the right dose. In Ferrazzi's words, *"Today's kids... their social-media-driven upbringing will make them savants in some areas of relationship building, and idiots in others..."*

In a nutshell, social media outlets shouldn't be your primary sources of interaction, but should instead be places where you sync up with the global hive and points from which you maintain your connections, friendships, and relationships, which are based on personal and reciprocal interaction and trust, and ideally actual flesh-and-blood meetups, dinner parties, social events and other inherently human activities that allow for everything from eye contact to smelling someone's unique bacterial scent to sensing the invisible yet detectable pheromones they release.

Now don't get me wrong: you do not need to be an extroverted social butterfly who spends every evening hour of each weekday hopping from a baseball game to a charity event to a plant foraging meetup to a bridge club to a dinner party to reap these benefits. A number of studies have shown that your own internal subjective sense of connection, compassion or love suffice to protect your health, happiness and well-being. This means that rather than dropping everything to go attend every cocktail party and golf game you're invited to, it's OK instead to simply have a few close friends you can confide in, a daily gratitude practice in which you identify one person you can pray for, help or serve that day, and a weekly hobby or event in which you're around just a few people who you love and who love you.

Of course, I'm not going to just leave you with that. Instead, I have a few practical tips up my sleeve that have really enhanced my own ability to be able to surround myself with more love and to build social engagement and a sense of community.

6 Ways To Enhance Your Life & Longevity With Love

#1: Volunteer

Volunteering is a win-win for all parties involved. Those who receive your help will be grateful, and you'll fill your own life with more empathy, sympathy and love. Consider the following as ways you can start volunteering:

- *Care for your parents.* We live in a culture in which our parents and the elderly are often relegated to nursing homes and hospice. But in an ideal community, you'd sacrifice your time, space and money to bring your parents into your own home, the same as they did for you when you were a baby. Even if they're not living with you but they instead live close to you, you can drop by for coffee on a Saturday morning, mow their yard, or accompany them on a shopping trip.

- *Help a local school.* Educators are overworked and stressed, while the children at many institutions need role models and people who care about their lives and behavior. You can volunteer to read stories to elementary school students, monitor outdoor activities, chaperone field trips or even work with a local church or other charitable organization to ensure that poor children are able to get food on the weekends. In our community, this program is called "Bite2Go" and each week a volunteer from my church drops off boxes of food at the school.

- *Visit a nursing home to sing or to visit.* As I alluded to above, many nursing homes are turned into dumping grounds for older people whose families are gone or are unavailable, and many residents are desperate for conversation and connections with outside individuals. Pick up the phone and call a local home, asking if you can come by and play guitar or piano, sing, help cook, take folks on walks or simply visit. I often visit local nursing homes with my twin boys to sing and play guitar, and when I was growing up, homes would often allow myself and my siblings, along with our parents, to take nursing home residents to local venues such as the fair or the symphony. Similarly, hospitals also have many volunteer opportunities that include everything from sitting with patients to working with children to food service and pushing wheelchairs.

- *Coach a sport.* Many kids don't get the opportunity to participate in sports because there aren't enough coaches or assistants. Even if you're not a "pro" in the sport for which you choose to help, you can volunteer to coach for your own child's team or any local youth sports team. I've personally done this for Valley Boys & Girls' Club basketball, my local University sports camps programs, and my twin boys' sports teams.

- *Tutor.* From children to adults, there are robust opportunities in most communities to tutor students, teach literacy, cooking, sewing or home repairs to adults, teach English and even help with classes on computers and other skills (the latter is especially needed and appreciated in the senior community).

- *Deliver meals.* I grew up in a family that delivered "Meals on Wheels" to the homeless, the unemployed, the elderly and the poor each week. Many communities have programs like this, and some even allow you to help with the meal prep.

- *Become a docent.* A what? A docent is a trained guide who leads visitors through facilities such as museums, art galleries, presidential libraries, aquariums, zoos, and universities. Your docent "training" is usually provided for free by these institutions.

- *Serve your own neighborhood.* In our modern era of digital connections, it's now all-too-common for neighbors not to know one another (can you name all your neighbors?), since you can easily join a Facebook group that contains avatars with far more similar interests than the person who lives next door to you. But neighborhood barbecues and beautification projects, helping your neighbor mow or shovel snow, and participation in a neighborhood organization builds a strong sense of local community.

#2: Dinner Parties

My friend Jayson Gaignard, author of the book *Mastermind Dinners: Build Lifelong Relationships by Connecting Experts, Influencers,* and Linchpins has built his entire career around connecting people and networks via hosting what he called "Mastermind Dinners." Of course, Keith Ferrazzi's classic networking book *Never Eat Alone,* which you've already discovered in this chapter, highlights the importance of convening people over food, but Jayson has truly perfected the process. He typically organizes dinners of eight to sixteen people in various major cities across the US and Canada (although he recommends six for the most intimate "sweet spot" if you really want people to get to know one another), and encourages that if we do the same, we should think carefully about who we invite to these meals and look for uncommon commonalities that make it more likely the guests will resonate with one another. The book goes into far more detail, and I'd highly recommend you give it a read, but ultimately, a huge amount of community-building power lies in the simple act of throwing a dinner about once a month for the purpose of reconnecting old ties, connecting people who should know each other and connecting with people who you've meant to connect with for a long time.

#3: Meetups

One way to meet new people, to make friends or practice your social skills, is through "Meetups", which are typically organized over the internet, but result in flesh-and-blood people being brought together for everything from hiking to tennis to business networking and beyond. At the moment, the most popular and well-known site for this is Meetup.com, a website on which you can create a group, which costs a small amount of money, or join a group, which is free. It's free to join and go to events, but costs money if you want to form a group yourself. Reddit.com is another decent place to find meetups for people located in your city, as are a growing number of apps that include Skout, Excuses to Meet, Hey! Vina and Wiith. I'm currently a member of a plant foraging meetup (if we all die of mushroom poisoning, at least we die together) and a singer-songwriter meetup. Even if you go to a meetup just one time, you're still likely to connect with at least one similarly interested person who winds up becoming a friend.

#4: Church

When it comes to forming deep, personal, meaningful relationships with like-minded individuals who share a belief in the importance of characteristics such as peace, love, joy, purpose and belief in a higher power, there's not a more likely place than a church to fit that need, and to also provide you with an avenue to further explore the benefits of caring for your spirit. Granted, I'll admit that the modern church has a scarred and sometimes sordid past of extreme judgmentalism and abuse, but I think you'll find that at your local neighborhood place of worship you're more likely to find a great deal of love and care from others than you are at a dogmatic or socially intolerable scenario.

Even though I'm a Christian, as an introvert I have personally struggled in the past with attending church. Frankly, I'd rather be wandering through the forest on an awe-inspiring hike while listening to a sermon or speaking with God. But I've also discovered that I can't just navigate through life as a spiritual lone wolf without the encouragement, collective worship, volunteer opportunities, and church community that is defined by the Greek word "Koinonia" which literally translated means communion, joint participation and the state of uplifting fellowship and unity that can and should exist within a church. There's even a growing body of evidence that demonstrates both physical and psychological benefits of singing in a choir (admittedly there are many choirs and singing groups you can join outside of a church, but having a large organized group of people to sing with is just one more benefit of being in a church).

#5: Renewing Forsaken Family Relationships

A recent research project at the UK's University of Cambridge called "Stand Alone", showed that family estrangements that arise from partner choices, addiction, illness, inheritance arguments and divorce are incredibly common, with estrangement from fathers being the most common and tending to last an average of almost eight years. Estrangements between brothers lasts 7.7 years, sisters around 7.4 years and mothers at 5.5 years. That's a large chunk of time to, as the Bible verse says, "allow the sun to go down on your anger", and the stress, tension and emotional pain that accompanies these estrangements are definitely not a healthy state of vibrational energy at which to exist.

I've certainly had my own fair share of family conflicts: bitterness against my father for not being more present and for divorcing my mother, resent against my mother for being overprotective during my childhood, judgement against my sister for marrying someone I initially thought was "the wrong guy," frustration towards my brothers for not being more responsible with their lives and families - the list goes on and on. I'll admit that it even feels therapeutic to tell you about these personal issues of mine, and I'll admit this also: I'm not perfect, I'm still working on mending each of those relationships and I'm very much responsible for creating many of these family rifts in my life.

Interestingly, the Australian documentary *Look Me In The Eye,* actually explored what happens when real families who are estranged make attempts to reconnect with each other and restore broken relationships. It shows that estranged family members often have an uneasy relationship with change, find change to be difficult, and therefore find that resolving estrangement feels out of their control. This is certainly the case with me: I'm a creature of habit who often becomes frustrated about things that I perceive to be outside my control and gives up on what seems to be outside my control. So how can you re-establish and mend broken family relationships? Here are a few tips:

- Reach out to the family member (and note that these same strategies should be applied to any broken relationship in your life - not just family members). Nothing is likely to happen unless you make that initial contact. Chances are high that multiple attempts will be necessary, and chances are also high that you'll be more successful picking up the phone or traveling to resolve issues face-to-face, vs. communicating via often impersonal emails and emoticons.

- Interestingly, and related to the last tip above, the method of re-connection they used in the documentary Look Me In The Eye was direct eye contact, which was based on neuroscience research showing that direct eye contact significantly helps people to communicate in difficult circumstances. So there's yet another reason to be present personally when resolving conflicts.

- Communicate clearly. Acknowledge the issues that are unresolved by naming them (e.g. "I've been angry with you for the past four years since you married Gwyneth, who I felt really wasn't the right person for you and messed up your life"). Lay all the cards out on the table.

- Consider family counseling with a pastor, counselor or psychiatry professional, especially if complex, thorny and unresolved issues threaten to remain, or if trying to solve the issue yourself doesn't seem to be producing any progress.

- Understand that it may take significant time, effort, sacrifice and, well, love to rebuild trust and respect.

#6: Reclaim Real Conversation

During a late night TV interview with Conan O' Brian, Louis C.K., (as controversial as the comedian is), said this about children communicating via the internet and smartphones:

> "And they don't look at people when they talk to them and they don't build empathy. You know, kids are mean, and it's 'cause they're trying it out. They look at a kid and they go, "you're fat," and then they see the kid's face scrunch up and they go, "oh, that doesn't feel good to make a person do that." But they got to start with doing the mean thing. But when they write "you're fat," then they just go, "mmm, that was fun, I like that."

Louis makes a good point: not only are digital conversations less empathetic, most likely due in large part to the loss of eye contact and other important physical elements of human interaction you learned earlier in this chapter, but it's also easier to hide your true emotions behind the invisibility of internet interaction, feel less guilty or less hesitant about trolling or making offensive remarks, and to engage in fake, inauthentic conversation.

The opposite of this would be what author Sherry Turkle in her book *Reclaiming Conversation* would refer to as real, authentic, personal conversation.

In her book, Sherry notes that it's all too common for the dinner table to fall silent as children compete with phones for their parents' attention, for you to not say a peep to the person sitting next to you on the airplane because both of you are sucked into the screen, and for two phones to be slapped on the center of the table in between spouses or lovers on a date. Heck, I've personally even developed the skill to be able to text message one person while conversing with and looking into the eyes of another person - an extreme example of being disconnected and halfway connected all at once.

Sherry points out that the case for conversation begins with conversations of solitude and self-reflection. They are endangered: these days, always connected, we see loneliness as a problem that technology should solve. Afraid of being alone, we rely on other people to give us a sense of ourselves, and our capacity for empathy and relationship suffers.

Back to Louis C.K.'s interview with Conan O' Brian (I'll link to a full video of the interview on the resources page for this chapter). Louis notes our propensity to grab our phones at any given time when we begin to feel loneliness creep in on us, including while in our vehicles:

> "Just that knowledge that it's all for nothing and that you're alone. You know it's down there. And sometimes when things clear away you are not watching it, you are in your car and you start going "oh, no, here comes that I'm alone like it starts to visit you". You know, just the sadness...Life is tremendously sad just by being in it, and so you're driving and then you go ah-ah-ah that's why we text and drive. I look around pretty much 100% of people driving are texting. And they are killing, everybody's murdering each other with their cars."

But as you've already discovered, this quest to be constantly connected is increasing, not decreasing loneliness (and also making the average highway a very dangerous place to be!) because technology interaction simply can't replace real, flesh-and-blood, face-to-face interaction. This form of real conversation builds empathy, friendship, love, learning, and productivity, and the book *Reclaiming Conversation* argues that the most human and humanizing thing that we can do is to engage in person-to-person conversation.

How? Here are a few tips, particularly focused around mealtimes, which I consider to be one of the best ways to engage meaningfully and the best times to "reclaim" conversation (much to the chagrin of frequent five-day water fasting enthusiasts!).

- **Reconfigure Your Phone:** If your email, text messages, and social media apps ping you every time a notification rolls in, you've not only lost control of your day, but also the ability to be able to engage in real conversation without being distracted. Your routine and your conversations now depend not on your schedule, but on whatever's happening on your phone. But as you no doubt know, Android, iOS and individual apps all have settings to stem the flow of alerts, buzzes, and rings. Every single notification on my phone is off, my phone is in silent mode and if I'm on a date or having dinner with the family, the phone is in airplane mode or Do Not Disturb mode. There is absolutely no need for you to be ripped away from a deep, meaningful conversation every time a Facebook friend tags you in a post. In extreme cases of smartphone addiction and lack of self control, you can even install addiction-breaking apps such as AppDetox, which lets you set limits on the time you spend inside individual apps; Flipd, which focuses on blocking access to certain apps for set periods of time; Onward, which allows you to track how often you use your phone and individual apps, set up rules for limiting phone use, and even have an expert give you personalized coaching to help break your tech addiction; and Forest (my favorite), which takes a slightly different approach by gamifying the process of easing you away from phone distractions. In Forest, you plant a seed, which eventually grows into a tree as long as you don't navigate away from the app. If you ditch Forest during the growth period to check Facebook or surf Safari, your tree will die. Admittedly, this sounds gimmicky, but is actually a very effective and dare-I-say meditative way of avoiding the temptations rife within your phone.

- **Play Table Topics:** Whether I'm on a date with my wife or at home with my family, a potent and fun way to completely forget the existence of my phone is to play a game of "Table Topics", also known as "Dinner Conversations", in which each person at the table asks a question from an official Table Topics card game, a Table Topics app (ironic, but can be used with the phone in airplane mode) or a printed list of Table Topics that include questions such as "If you could have any superhero sitting here at dinner with us, who would you choose and why?" or

"What was the scariest decision you made in the past year?" or "If your house were on fire and you could put three objects in a backpack before you rushed out, what would you choose and why?". You get the idea. It may seem silly that you'd need your conversation topics chosen for you to engage in "real conversation", but I and my family have spent many valuable minutes at dinner laughing and learning more about one another with this approach, and often the questions rabbit-hole into even deeper conversations.

- **Share Gratitude Journals:** In Chapter 10, you discovered the power of gratitude and the three most important questions you can journal each morning. At our house, we bring our journals to the dinner table and discuss what we wrote. When a family of four, or even a group of two, embark upon a conversation about what they are grateful for, what they discovered in the morning's reading and who they helped, prayed for or served that day, it can lead to deep and meaningful conversation that can often last for the entire dinner.

- **Taste the Food:** Allow me to point out a painfully obvious fact: when you're at a meal you are eating - often filling your face with wonderful and interesting molecules that are highly conducive to conversation. So why not share your opinions of a meal's taste, texture or presentation? Why not discuss the culinary expertise put into the food (which can work when at a fancy restaurant, but may not be so handy when eating Aunt Edna's macaroni-and-cheese)? Why not sip the wine, flavor-taste the salt or try a set of new spices and discuss what your brain experiences? Just last night at our house, my wife, twin boys and I spent nearly twenty minutes tasting and trying three different bottles of olive oil and - similar to a wine tasting - commenting on the notes, the flavors, the aromas and the subtle details of each oil, and what we liked best about it. The bonus of this strategy? You tend to eat less and become fuller faster because you're actually savoring your food!

And finally, should all else fail, you can rely upon Jayson Gaignard's trick that he reveals at just about every one of his Mastermind Dinners I've attended: all phones get piled up onto the middle of the table in airplane mode or off, and the first person to reach for their device pays for dinner.

Summary

Ultimately, having a great job, being fit, living in a nice home, or any other creature comfort can all be for naught if loneliness, sadness, inflammation, high blood pressure and accelerated aging are all occurring due to lack of friendships, social relationships, community, charity and love in your life. But you're now equipped to include these important components into your own life. Finally, be sure to consider reading the following books within the next year:

- *Never Eat Alone*

- *Reclaiming Conversation*

- *Mastermind Dinners*

- *I'd Like You More If You Were More Like Me*

- *The Power of Introverts* (if you are indeed an introvert or suspect you are)

This week, take a loved one or friend on a date, an adventure, a walk or just a quick meal or chat, but leave your phone behind. Not "off" in your pocket, but truly forsaken back at home or your office. Notice how this changes the conversation or experience. At this point in Fit Soul, you can have become accustomed to a bit of spiritual weight training. In the next several chapters, I'm going to put a bit more weight onto the bar for you, so to speak and tackle some incredibly meaningful and life-changing topics. The next chapter, though it may seem oriented towards the male population, which is somewhat true, is a chapter I still encourage you to read if you are a mother, a sister, a woman or any member of the female population with a man in her life. You will benefit.

For resources, references, links and additional reading and listening material for this chapter, visit FitSoulBook.com/Chapter6.

CHAPTER VII

BE A MAN

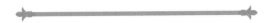

I lived much of my life as a boy.

Deep down inside, driving my masochistic forays into twenty years of obstacle course and adventure racing, triathlons, sporting competitions, and brutal workouts was a deep-seated desire to prove to the world that I was a man.

At home, driven by a fear of rejection and resentment by my wife and children, and a preference for people-pleasing, I was loose-handed in discipline or "laying down the law" in any sort of authoritarian fashion. God forbid I would ever be remembered as some kind of tyrant or dictator of the home, so it must be far safer to simply be a likable pushover of a father, right? As a result, my role in the home was as a bit of a Homer Simpson-esque buffoon, a jolly and joking yet ultimately feeble Peter of the Family Guy cartoon, or Phil Dunphy of the Modern Family sitcom.

For years, I considered it a noble act to elevate my wife's status in the home to matriarchal Queen mother and caretaker of the household, yet this simultaneously allowed me to step into the shadows while allowing her to bear the burden of everything from breaking up arguments amongst our boys to ensuring the family was in time for church on Sundays to planning out the family's weekend activities. She was the Queen while I was the happy-go-lucky boyish jester whose presence in the household was more of a third son to her rather than a rock, a foundation, a father, a leader, and a king. After all, I figured it's far better for dad to be "cool" and accepted by his kids than to take on the responsibility of being a strong and inspirational patriarch of the family.

I was a weakling who shirked leadership.

I was afraid of being judged by my family.

I was amiable and charming, yet fragile, delicate, and soft.

But over the past few months, I have been observing the world around me and dwelling upon the way I was "leading" my family and experienced a stark realization: I needed to grow up. Permanent adolescence is a plague upon our society and our families that is threatening to unravel the quilt of culture in the very manner we are now witnessing. You're about to discover why, and what you can do about it—so pay attention (especially you, fellas).

OUR FATHERLESS WORLD

When it comes to the way that the world perceives the ideal father, times have certainly changed, haven't they?

For example, while I've never been much of a television and pop culture enthusiast, I have seen old American TV programs from the 40s, 50s, and 60s, such as "Father Knows Best" or "Leave It to Beaver," both of which—despite their often unrealistic portrayal of the perfect, idealized, nuclear family—depict relatively respectable father figures who lead their families in a strong, responsible and respectable manner. Next came the 70s, where fathers began to be portrayed much like the loudmouthed, uneducated bigot Archie Bunker of "All in the Family."

Then over the years leading up to our current era, Hollywood's portrayal of a father devolved into the Homer Simpson, the Peter Griffin, and the Phil Dunphy— buffoonish and irresponsible fathers who are largely clowns, pushovers, and weaklings.

Unfortunately, the modern household father has fared no better than the Hollywood father. Not only are fathers more inspired by these type of television portrayals to be likable, funny friends who call their kids "bud," but they also tend to be present on the smartphone while relatively absent in their children's' lives, able to escape family life via workaholism enabled by a hyperconnected home-office scenario, loose-handed with discipline in fear that a social worker may come knocking on the door asking about 7am burpees in the driveway, and stricken with the angst of possibly being depicted as sexist, chauvinistic, dogmatic, or any other negative term used to describe a dad who dares to be a strong, hard, dependable, manly, male figure.

Just check out the link I have on the resources page for this chapter to listen to the shock and awe response of many of the children immersed in my friend Joe De Sena's recent bootcamp for kids he organized at his home in Vermont and described on the

Joe Rogan show, and read some of the comments of his description. God forbid children be pushed by older male figures, and exposed to hardship, cold, lifting heavy objects, getting up early, and learning to be tough! I highly doubt the same response would have taken place if adolescent rites of passage were woven into our culture as they had been for eons of time, but frankly, most boys never even have an opportunity to experience this ceremonial recognition of their passage into manhood and subsequent societal responsibilities of protecting and providing for their family, their village, their community, and their country.

This modern backslide into male weakness is accompanied by the same censorship of true, honorable manly strength that got former president Theodore Roosevelt fired from his Sunday School teacher position. While at Harvard, Roosevelt actually taught Sunday school at a local church, but apparently he was too much of a muscular Christian (read more on his flavor of muscular Christianity in the ArtOfManliness link on the resources page for this chapter) for the church body. Case in point: One day a boy came to class with a black eye. He admitted he had been in a fight, on Sunday, no less. A much bigger boy had been pinching his sister and he got into a fistfight with him.

> *"You did perfectly right," said Roosevelt and proceeded to give him a dollar. The church vestrymen thought this was going too far and subsequently removed Roosevelt from his position as Sunday school teacher. (These days, I imagine Roosevelt would not only have been removed, but also vilified and canceled on all his social media accounts, and lambasted by women's rights organizations for implying that small women somehow need to be defended by their older brothers.)*

But it gets worse. In many households today, not only are fathers not being the kings, leaders, and men they need to be, but there is often no father presence whatsoever, which leads to an even more serious problem.

See, children in fatherless homes begin life at a significant disadvantage. For example, statistics show that the majority of prison inmates come from broken families and that those broken families are most often fatherless families. Furthermore, when fathers aren't present, an entity must step in to take the place of protector and provider. Sadly, that is most often not the local church or parish stepping up to the plate to care for the widows and fatherless, nor a grandparent or other loving family member, but instead, the government.

In other words, fathers aren't present. So government welfare has stepped in to replace the role of a father. Boys raised in such a home grow up without a rock, a foundation and a male leader, and thus rinse, wash, and repeat a vicious cycle— venturing out into the world without a strong sense of responsibility or rite of passage into manhood, knocking up a few ladies, producing more unwanted babies, and propagating a continued cycle of aborted babies and/or fatherless homes.

If it were classified as a disease, fatherlessness would be an epidemic worthy of attention as a national emergency. More than 20 million children live in a home without the presence of a father. Millions more children have fathers who are physically present, yet emotionally absent. You can check out the resources page for this chapter to read plenty more statistics on the sad extent of fatherlessness.

In his book, *Hearts of the Fathers,* author Charles Crismier notes that many children today who grow up in a fatherless home lack a *"God-ordered earthly anchor for soul security"*, noting that *"It is well known but seldom discussed, whether in the church house or the White House, that fatherlessness lies at the root of nearly all of the most glaring problems that plague our modern, now post-Christian life."* He goes on to point out that children living in female-headed homes have a poverty rate of 48 percent, more than four times the rate for children living in homes with their fathers and mothers.

Another author, Paul Vitz, in his book *Faith of the Fatherless: The Psychology of Atheism,* writes that—in stark contrast to the fruits of a fatherless home—strong spiritual leaders often had remarkably positive and present fathers or father figures. In one television interview, he states: *"I would say the biggest problem in the country is the breakdown of the family, and the biggest problem in the breakdown in the family is the absence of the father. Our answer is to recover the faith, particularly for men, and we'll recover fatherhood. And if we recover fatherhood, we'll recover the family. If we recover the family, we'll recover our society."*

In his recent essay noting the sad state of the church in America and its failure to step up for clear constitutional rights during the COVID quarantine, Doug Wilson says: *"The reason why the streets of Chicago are filled with violence is fatherlessness. The reason why so many young people flock to the false allure of socialism is fatherlessness. The reason why there is massive contempt for our institutions is fatherlessness, and the reason why our institutions have become so contemptible is fatherlessness."*

But the fact is, your own home does not need to be fatherless, physically absent of a patriarch, or without the presence of a male figurehead to experience the same issues.

To destroy your legacy, continue to make our nation's families weak, continue to propagate the cycle of poverty and violence, and continue to create a culture of Homer Simpsons, Peter Griffins, and Phil Dunphys, all you need to do is keep being a boy. Your home simply needs to have you, the supposed father, mentally and spiritually absent: a likable, soft-boned buffoon.

How To Be A Man

So what can you as a father do to break this vicious cycle, become a true reflection of the ultimate man that God created you to be, and create a culture of strong, responsible males who will step up for their rights and protect and provide for their families?

I have three suggestions for you.

1. Be a king.

Quit operating in your home as the court jester. Sure, you can be likable, amicable, and a pleasant, kind and joyful presence in your household, but don't take it so far that your children or wife don't take you seriously because you haven't a drop of stoicism or seriousness in your body.

So what is a king, exactly?

Just look up the definition of king in a dictionary...

...a male sovereign or monarch...

...a man who holds by life tenure, and usually by hereditary right...

...a person or thing preeminent in its class...

...or here's the way I like to think of it: Picture Aslan, the great Lion of C.S. Lewis's *Chronicles Of Narnia.* Aslan is depicted as the King of Beasts, the son of the Emperor-Over-the-Sea, and the King above all High Kings in Narnia. He is awe-inspiring and a bit frightening, but unquestionably benevolent and kind, with unmatched power and unlimited goodness. That is the king you should aspire to be.

Or consider the words of Robert Greene from his book *48 Laws Of Power,* in which Law 34 commands those who seek power to "Be Royal in Your Own Fashion – Act Like a King To Be Treated Like One".

Greene explains: *"The way you carry yourself will often determine how you are treated: In the long run, appearing vulgar or common will make people disrespect you. For a king respects himself and inspires the sentiment in others. By acting regally and confident of your powers, you make yourself seem destined to wear a crown."*

So act royally if you want to be treated royally and taken seriously. Be sober, be confident, and command respect. If you plan to step up as the king of your family, begin to act like an actual king. How does a king act? Read Proverbs 31: 3-9, in which King Lemuel dictates to his son what it takes to be a true king:

> *"Listen, my son! Listen, son of my womb! Listen, my son, the answer to my prayers! Do not spend your strength on women, your vigor on those who ruin kings. It is not for kings, Lemuel— it is not for kings to drink wine, not for rulers to crave beer, lest they drink and forget what has been decreed, and deprive all the oppressed of their rights. Let beer be for those who are perishing, wine for those who are in anguish! Let them drink and forget their poverty and remember their misery no more. Speak up for those who cannot speak for themselves, for the rights of all who are destitute. Speak up and judge fairly; defend the rights of the poor and needy."*

A king must remain alert and in possession of all his faculties at all times. A king cannot afford to let himself fall into a stupor that will erode the respect of others and have devastating consequences should an attack of the enemy occur. A king cannot afford to be careless and sloppy.

Titus 2:2 in the Bible teaches that: *"Older men are to be sober-minded, dignified, self-controlled, sound in faith, in love, and in steadfastness..."*

So are you such an older man, a king, and an inspirational figurehead for your family, or are you still a sober-less, undignified, weak-willed, faithless boy?

Do you need to quit smoking weed and crashing on the couch at night?

Do you need to stop sucking down your "microdoses" of plant medicine and wine and crawling into your basement man cave to escape your responsibilities?

Do you need to begin to speak up for what you know is right and a full expression of your true, authentic self, rather than who you think the world expects you to be or what an unconstitutional silly government clothing, living and shopping mandate being shoved down your throat dictates?

Then do it. Be royal. Be stoic. Be taken seriously. Stand up for what you know is right. Be a king.

2. Be a leader.

Quit lazily allowing your wife (as I did for so many years)—no matter how strong a woman she may be—to step into a position of leadership that places undue stress upon her shoulders and removes responsibility from yours. It is your position as a father to create a culture in your family that inspires respect, love, joy, peace, and trust.

What does being a strong leader of your home look like?

Take responsibility for your household and don't be - as Doug Wilson describes in his book *Father Hunger* - just one more person living in this household: just one more of the roommates. Don't be "a boy who shaves". The opposite of being a "boy who shaves" is true masculinity, which is the glad assumption of sacrificial responsibility. A man who assumes responsibility is learning masculinity, and a culture that encourages men to take responsibility is a culture that is a friend to masculinity.

Establish family values and create a culture in your household by leading your family in spiritual disciplines such as meditation, prayer, gratitude journaling, clear identification of purpose statements, and the other practices I teach you about in this book.

Be present, mentally, physically, and emotionally. Put down your phone already. Look your children and wife in the eyes. No good leader is an absent leader.

Create traditions and build a legacy. Remember: you aren't just raising your children, you're raising your children's children, and everything you do in your home—from how you wake to how you eat to how you speak to how you compete to how you create—will all be observed and copied very closely by your children and future generations.

Create calendars, systems, and accountability for your home. Use Google Calendar, use an app or platform like Habitory to hold the family accountable in their daily practices, set up schedules so that family dinners become prioritized and begin to think of yourself (not your wife!) as a manager and chief operations officer of the home, and don't just show up where you're told. Instead, you decide who shows up where and when.

Consider a rite of passage for your boys. Options abound.I delve into rites of passage on the podcast I'll link to on the resources page for this chapter. Many organizations, often in the realm of wilderness survival and nature immersion, exist to systematize the process of a rite of passage for a young man. Begin by Googling a term such as "wilderness rite of passage NAME OF YOUR CITY for boys." My own boys will have multiple solo, ego-dissolving days in the wilderness between the ages of 13 and 15, accompanied by a ceremonial coming of age led by the people I trust at Twin Eagles Wilderness School. Following that rite of passage, they'll also experience their first responsibly facilitated use of plant medicines to further dissolve the ego and prepare them to become kings, leaders, fathers, and husbands for life. The rite of passage for your own boys doesn't need to be the same as mine, but hopefully, this gives you some ideas of where to start.

And finally, lead with love. You are not a soulless dictator. You are not a grumpy general who barks orders each morning. You are not a ruthless authoritarian. You gaze at others deeply in the eye, you smile kindly, you hug, you snuggle, you prepare wonderful nourishing meals, you teach with patience, you sacrifice time to be fully present, and you respect your children and your wife. Remember: be an Aslan.

As Doug Wilson says in his excellent book *"Father Hunger: Why God Calls Men to Love and Lead Their Families:"*

> *"What are fathers called to? Fathers give. Fathers protect. Fathers bestow. Fathers yearn and long for the good of their children. Fathers delight. Fathers sacrifice. Fathers are jovial and open-handed. Fathers create abundance, and if lean times come they take the leanest portion themselves and create a sense of gratitude and abundance for the rest. Fathers love birthdays and Christmas because it provides them with yet another excuse to give some more to the kids. When fathers say no, as good fathers do from time to*

time, it is only because they are giving a more subtle gift, one that is a bit more complicated than a cookie. They must also include among their gifts things like self-control and discipline and a work ethic, but they are giving these things, not taking something else away just for the sake of taking. Fathers are not looking for excuses to say no. Their default mode is not no."

So be the father and husband who makes wild love to your wife at night, wakes early in the morning to bake your family chocolate chip cookies for the evening family dinner, then rips your boys out of bed to go lift heavy kettlebells in the garage and drag sandbags up and down the driveway—followed by dirty, sweaty bear hugs afterward. But don't be the father and husband who stays absent and distracted with "noble" email and social media work all day, then gathers the family round Netflix in the basement in the evening so they can eat takeout while you have an excuse to dink on your phone some more as they're distracted by their own giant screen.

3. Be a man of God.

Finally, to be a true leader and true king, you must seek your own spiritual fitness diligently and daily. In *"Father Hunger,"* Wilson also says:

"... men must seek to be Christians first. If they love Jesus Christ more than mother or father, or wife, or sons, or daughters, then they will be in fellowship with the source of all love. If they make an idol out of any one of their family members, then they are out of fellowship with the source of all love — meaning that the "idol" is short-changed. A man's wife receives far more love when she is number 2 after God than she would if she were number 1. A man's children will be fathered diligently when they are loved in the context of a much greater love."

In other words, you must seek and experience God's love to be able to give full love to your family. You must steep yourself in God's word and be in full union with Him daily.

How is that going for you?

Are you caring for the one component of your human existence that is so often shriveled, shrunken, and neglected inside? If not, read Chapter 10, then, in addition to daily immersion in the Bible, delve into books such as:

- *Celebration of Discipline: The Path to Spiritual Growth* by **Richard Foster**

- *Spiritual Disciplines for the Christian Life* by **Donald S. Whitney**

- *Spiritual Disciplines Handbook* by **Adele A. Calhoun**

- *The Jesuits Guide to (Almost) Everything: A Spirituality for Real Life* by **James Martin, SJ**

- *Solitude: A Philosophical Encounter* by **Philip Koch**

That ought to be enough to get you started in your path to spiritual health and becoming a man of God. Now take action. Once the kids are in bed, turn off your phone at night and start reading books like those above. That's what I've done for the past four years and it's been absolutely transformative.

Summary

Fortunately, we have a complete manual for being a father in an increasingly fatherless world: the Bible—and I'd be remiss not to finish with what we can learn from the world's only written source of absolute truth. What does the Bible tell us about being a father who reflects the full greatness of God the Father? Plenty! As a matter of fact, fathers are so important in the Bible (beginning with God the Father) that the words "father," "fathers," and "forefathers" appear 1,573 times.

Psalm 23:1-6 says: "*The Lord is my shepherd; I shall not want. He makes me lie down in green pastures. He leads me beside still waters. He restores my soul. He leads me in paths of righteousness for his name's sake. Even though I walk through the valley of the shadow of death, I will fear no evil, for you are with me; your rod and your staff, they comfort me. You prepare a table before me in the presence of my enemies; you anoint my head with oil; my cup overflow...*"

The Lord is our shepherd, and we as fathers should be the same for our family. You should want to be the father who can walk your own children through fear, through death, through shadows, and through evil, then train them up to be that same kind of shepherding father.

Proverbs 3:11-12 says: *"My son, do not despise the Lord's discipline or be weary of his reproof, for the Lord reproves him whom he loves, as a father the son in whom he delights."*, Ephesians 6:4: *"Fathers, do not provoke your children to anger, but bring them up in the discipline and instruction of the Lord."*, Colossians 3:21: *"Fathers, do not provoke your children, lest they become discouraged."* and Psalm 103:13: *"As a father shows compassion to his children, so the Lord shows compassion to those who fear him."*

So we are to be firm rocks who provide discipline, but always in kindness, compassion, and love—because we delight in our children and wish them the very best. As you look to Scripture for patterns of masculinity, you will find them manifested perfectly in the life of Jesus, who set the ultimate pattern for love and courage in living out the ideal Hero's Journey that I describe in Chapter 9.

Beyond the Bible, there are other resources besides those I have already mentioned above that I recommend to you and encourage you to read if you want to continue in your evolution to becoming a true man, a king, a father, and a leader in your home—including *Be A Man! Becoming the Man God Created You to Be* by Larry Richards and *Future Men: Raising Boys to Fight Giants* by Doug Wilson (who wrote the equally good *Father Hunger* cited earlier). In addition, visit BenGreenfieldFitness.com/boystomen to access an Amazon list I created two years ago. It contains several other titles that I'm reading with my own boys—titles I chose to make boys great men and men greater men.

How about you? Do you plan to step up to the plate and accept the responsibility of your role as a father, a leader, and a king? How are you rising to the occasion for your family and being a rock and a foundation for your wife and children? If you are a woman, how do you plan to support the men or boys in your life to rise to their own role as fathers, leaders and kings? If you have found yourself struggling with motivation, meaning or direction as you tackle the questions I'm asking you at the end of each chapter, then pay heed to the next chapter, because you're going to get the key for unlocking boundless energy at your beck and call, all day long.

For resources, references, links and additional reading and listening material for this chapter, visit FitSoulBook.com/Chapter7.

How to Find your Purpose in Life

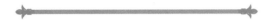

In Chapter 2, I described the vast importance of Presence, and how the growing awareness of the magic of Presence influenced my own retooling of my purpose statement for life.

But how exactly *does* one form a purpose statement, and why is that important anyways?

That's exactly what you're about to discover.

Let's start here...

In my book *Boundless: Upgrade Your Brain, Optimize Your Body & Defy Aging*, I describe in one chapter what I refer to as "my most potent tip for increasing your energy vibration and the vibrations of all people around you". That tip was this...

...identify your purpose in life and enable yourself to achieve that unique purpose to the very best of your ability, all while loving God and loving others as fully as possible with that purpose.

See, when it comes to being happy and living a long time, it's not your 48th ayahuasca trip, relentless pursuit of six-pack abs, crushing a new workout personal record, finally discovering the perfect diet, engaging in free-wheeling polyamory and open relationships, or any other recent infatuation of the health, wellness, and longevity movement I have witnessed so many times.

All flesh and blood is like a plant that eventually withers and dies. Just look around. The fastest track athlete will eventually be defeated by muscle loss, neural degradation, and arthritis. The most beautiful supermodel in the world will not be on the cover of the Sports Illustrated Swimsuit Issue when she's ninety-seven years old. Even wealthy, powerful CEOs who can throw money at nearly every problem eventually get betrayed by their bodies and die.

Yep, we fade. We wither away. As 1 Peter 1:24 in the Bible says: *"All people are like grass, and all their glory is like the flowers of the field; the grass withers and the flowers fall."*

What is in fact contributing most to your energy vibrations at any given moment isn't your beauty or your fitness or your accomplishments, but your soul. Therein lies your ability to be, as the title of my last book alludes to, truly boundless. I even have a tattoo that I emblazoned onto the skin of my shoulder when I was just 20 years old. It's the Japanese Kanji symbol for Ki: which is also known as chi, soul, spirit, chakra and prana. It is the invisible, boundless life force that flows through all of us. Caring for this all-encompassing energy of my body and fueling it with the spiritual disciplines and union with God is how I now live my life.

See, true and lasting happiness is not achieved by external circumstances, nor your thoughts, nor your intentions, nor even your feelings, but rather your soul. In his book *Soul Keeping,* author John Ortberg defines the soul as that aspect of your whole being that correlates, integrates and enlivens everything else. He writes that we all have two worlds: an outer world that is visible and public and obvious, and an inner world that may be chaotic and dark, or may be gloriously beautiful.

In the end, the outer world fades, and all you are then left with is your inner world.

But ironically, the more obsessed we are with ourselves, our fitness, our cognitive performance, our finances, and our food, the more we tend to neglect our souls. When your soul is not centered and in the right place, you tend to define yourself by your accomplishments, your physical appearance, your title, or your social circles and friends. But then, when you lose any of these attachments, you tend to lose your identity. I've experienced this myself when I've gotten injured, sick, or had a poor race or workout and subsequently felt like I was losing my happiness and transitioning to a lower level of energy vibration because I was losing my shaky identity as an "athlete" or a "healthy person." Suddenly the emptiness of those shallow pursuits became distinctly magnified.

Perhaps this is why one of my favorite Bible verses, Mark 8:36, which I first introduced to you in the introduction of this book, says, *"What does it profit a man to gain the whole world and forfeit his soul?"*

So *how* do you connect with and care for your soul? I'll tell you how.

You must ask yourself: *What is the core part of you that you want folks to talk about at your funeral?*

In other words, what is your *purpose*?

If you're not clear on this, ask some people who know you pretty well, such as your immediate family or close friends, to describe to you why they think God placed you on this planet and what the unique skills and talents are that seem to flow naturally from you. Ask them what they think should be written on your gravestone. Ask them what they think your unique purpose is. I'll hazard a guess that it's not that you were the best exerciser, or that you ate an amazing, flawless diet, or that you had gorgeous skin, or that you made oodles of money.

But you can't stop there. It's not enough to simply identify your purpose (a process I'll teach you how to do shortly). To truly connect with and care for your soul, you must also connect with your inner self, and ask yourself this one question:

> *"What aspect of my life can I change today that will allow me to care for my soul so that I can identify and achieve that purpose?"*

Maybe it begins with a meditation practice. Maybe stepping into a church. Maybe mending a broken relationship. Maybe stopping to breathe and be present. Maybe dropping a relentless pursuit of a better body and brain and instead realizing that your approach has been horribly skewed and that to truly achieve deep, meaningful satisfaction in life, you must begin to care for the most important part of you that will exist for eternity and begin to share that discovery with the rest of the world by living your entire life based on your core purpose.

No matter what it is that must change, you'll find that you must often radically change your environment to radically change your habits. This might mean staying in bed an extra ten minutes to read your Bible or complete a gratitude journal, ditching the evening Netflix binge to spend time with God or your family, and taking a weekend day of rest and recovery to go and volunteer at a homeless shelter, neighbor's garden or soup kitchen rather than going on a 2-hour hike, playing catch-up with phone calls, or doing back-to-back workouts (an all-too-common Sunday habit of many of the fitness enthusiasts with whom I hang).

So let me ask you this: What is your purpose? And how alive is your soul so that you can identify and fuel that purpose? Now, take a deep breath in through your nose, and out through your mouth. Sense your spirit. Sense your soul. Feel it? It's there. It may be shriveled up and dry and neglected but it's there, ready for you to grow and nurture it. Take one more deep breath in through your nose, then smile and breathe out. You are an amazing soul. You are here for a purpose.

Are you now convinced that having a purpose is of pretty significant importance in your life? If so, and if you still need help identifying or developing your purpose and your personal why, then keep reading.

HOW TO FIND YOUR PURPOSE IN LIFE

So now we get down to brass tacks. How exactly does one identify their purpose in life?

I've studied up on this quite a bit, and there are plenty of purpose-finding materials and resources I've thoroughly read and reviewed, with some of my favorites including:

- *"Claim Your Power"* by **Mastin Kipp**

- *"Limitless"* by **Jim Kwik**

- *"Personality Isn't Permanent"* by **Benjamin Hardy**

- *"The Values Factor"* by **John DiMartini**

- *"Don't Waste Your Life"* by **John Piper**

- *"True North: Discover Your Authentic Leadership"* by **Bill George**

- *"The Lifebook Course"* by **Jon and Missy Butcher**

- **Websites such as** *Life Purpose Quiz, TheWhyStack.com, StartWithWhy.com,* **and** *WhyInstitute.com*

Geez. That's a lot of content about purpose. So do you now need to drop everything and spend the next three months of your life reading all that?

Maybe.

You'd probably come out the other side a better, more purposeful person.

But one area in which I think *I* can do *you* a convenient service is to succinctly distill into a few key tips what I personally learned from each of these books and websites, and what I see as recurring themes in most purpose-finding literature and resources like those cited above. I can guarantee that if you use the following steps and tips outlined below to identify your life purpose, you'll have harnessed 80% of the goodness from those resources above and be left with the *option* to delve into them in your own free time, if you so desire.

So here we go. I recommend that as you read the steps below, you sit down with a journal and jot down your replies with a pen or pencil and paper. If your'e reading on an e-reader, you may even want to print this section of Fit Soul and tuck it into a journal so you can step away from the computer, e-reader, or smartphone and into a different set and setting with few connections, distractions and notifications as you complete these exercises.

How To Find Your Purpose In Life, Step 1: What did you like to do when you were a kid?

You were born with a unique set of skills and talents; things you tend to be good at based on the way your brain is wired, the way your genetics are assembled, and the way your body is built. As a result of these nature-based traits, along with nurture-based influence from the family and households you grew up in, you likely tend to enjoy and be good at specific activities.

For example, I grew up absolutely loving reading books; writing stories; learning via documentaries, courses, and movies; teaching what I learned to others; singing songs; speaking in front of people; creating art and new ideas; and competing in sports and other games, such as chess and video games.

So my own personal purpose statement is, as you discovered in Chapter 2:

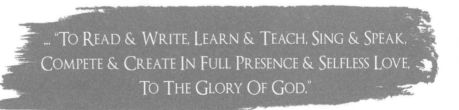

... "To Read & Write, Learn & Teach, Sing & Speak, Compete & Create In Full Presence & Selfless Love, To The Glory Of God."

See how that purpose statement weaves in many of the same activities that I loved when I was a child? Those are the activities that still ignite my joy and put me into a state of flow.

If you're a bit foggy about what you were actually like and what you enjoyed doing when you were a little boy or a little girl, then, if your parents or relatives who were close to you at that time are still alive, invite them out to dinner or a coffee. When you sit down with them, ask them one question:

"What was I like when I was a kid?"

That's it. Then prepare to sit back, listen, and take notes.

How To Find Your Purpose In Life, Step 2: What puts you "in the zone" now?

In the field of psychology, a flow state, also known as "being in the zone," is a mental state in which you are performing an activity in which you are fully immersed in a feeling of energized focus, full involvement, enjoyment, and presence during the process of engaging in that activity.

For example, if I sit down in front of a blank Word document on my computer and begin to write, my concept of time vanishes. I'll write for hours. Words just *flow* out of me. I don't think about food or drink, and I'm often oblivious to everything else going on around me, even if I'm in a busy coffee shop. I've always been wired that way. My wife, on the other hand, absolutely detests writing and would rather walk on a bed of nails than pen an essay. However, if you plant her in front of a blank canvas and give her a set of paintbrushes and a bit of oil or watercolor, she'll absolutely bloom with joy as she paints for hours on end, entering her own "zone" with a satisfied smile on her face (I, on the other hand, tend to painfully cringe as I forcefully attempt to "make art happen" on a blank canvas).

So what puts *you* in the zone at this point in your life? Writing? Art? Craftsmanship like woodworking or building something with your hands? Gardening? Exercise? Programming?

Identify those activities, and weave them into your purpose statement. I guarantee you'll find a great deal of overlap between those activities and what you enjoyed doing when you were a kid.

This may seem a bit redundant with the consideration of what you enjoyed doing when you were a kid and what puts you in the zone now, but it's important to take into account because if your purpose statement is built around those activities that naturally come easy to you, you'll be highly self-actualized as you live out that purpose statement. Self-actualized people are those who are significantly fulfilled, driven, and joyful in their day-to-day activities. For self-actualized people living out their true purpose in life, a day of work often feels like a day of play.

And guess what? There's absolutely nothing to be ashamed about if work comes easy to you. Often, we have a belief pattern, perhaps influenced by the traditional so-called Puritanical work ethic philosophy* that a day of work needs to be a day of drudge, drenched in blood, sweat, and tears; and we frequently believe that only at the end of a day of work can we take a deep sigh of relief and "play" (although we're typically so exhausted by the hard work that play is the equivalent of junk food binges, video games, and Netflix).

But, as Mark Twain said, if you *"find a job you enjoy doing, you will never have to work a day in your life."*

Others have shared Twain's thoughts. Here's what Stephen King has to say:

> *"Yes, I've made a great deal of dough from my fiction, but I never set a single word down on paper with the thought of being paid for it ... I have written because it fulfilled me. Maybe it paid off the mortgage on the house and got the kids through college, but those things were on the side--I did it for the buzz. I did it for the pure joy of the thing. And if you can do it for the joy, you can do it forever."*

Steve Jobs noted that:

> *"Your work is going to fill a large part of your life, and the only way to be truly satisfied is to do what you believe is great work. And the only way to do great work is to love what you do."*

Then there's Thomas Edison, who said:

> "I never did a day's work in my life, it was all fun."

You get the idea. Work can just flow from you. When it does, and when it feels like play, that's another sign you're living out your true purpose. Sure, there will be times when you experience what Steven Pressfield refers to as the "resistance"—rationalizing, fear and anxiety, distractions, the voice of an inner critic, and other elements that keep you from creating your authentic art (whatever that creation of art might be)—but this resistance doesn't indicate you're not living out your purpose. It's just a day-to-day temptation we all tend to face: a temptation towards laziness or fear of the unknown, failure, or embarrassment. Learn to identify the resistance to living your purpose, embrace the resistance as a sign that you're engaged in something impactful, then press on (and definitely read Steven's book *Do The Work!*).

*a quick note regarding the Puritanical work ethic. I don't mean to throw the Puritans under the bus. In the book, Exploring New England's Spiritual Heritage, author Garth Rosell describes how the Puritans were actually encouraged to identify their purpose in life with much prayer and reflection, to take into account their natural gifts and inclinations, to seek the advice and confirmation of their friends and family, and to consider the practical needs of the community in which they lived.

Interestingly, those who were gifted for and inclined to "sundry callings" (the equivalent of a blue-collar worker, such as farming, construction, horseshoeing, etc. - which in modern days could be the warehouse worker, firefighter, construction worker, custodian, etc.) must seek to discover which of these callings is "the best." Similarly, those who were privileged to study in what was called "the schools of the prophets" and at liberty to become school-masters, physicians, lawyers, or ministers were considered to have a special obligation to seek among these available options their very "best calling."

Regardless of what career was chosen by these Puritans, their callings were encouraged to conform to three basic principles. First, to serve the public good and to seek one another's welfare. Second, to have "gifts of body and mind" suitable to that calling (although they also believed rightly that when God calls a person to a particular task, he will also provide the appropriate gifts to fulfill it). Third, to be sure that calling is from God, by relying upon prayer, the guidance of the Bible, the counsel of friends, the encouragement of the community and the existence of an open door opportunity.

If that vocation was considered to be homely, boring or ordinary, they focused upon performing that task nonetheless to the glory of God and the good of others. After all, Jesus himself girded himself with a towel, and washed His disciples' feet. If a Puritan was anxious about whether or not their work was successful, they were encouraged to "cast their burden upon the Lord" and to find contentment whatever the circumstance.

So ultimately, while I don't think that work, especially working in our true purpose and calling, needs to be viewed as a daily drudge of sweat, blood and tears, I do agree with this Puritan philosophy that no matter what your work is, it should be chosen carefully according to your unique gifts and the counsel of God, friends and family, be done in full excellence, with a spirit of love towards others with no complaining, and finally, should "multiple purposes" be available to one, the best purpose is the one most highly suited to your gifts.

How To Find Your Purpose In Life, Step 4: Summarize your purpose into one single, succinct statement that you can memorize.

This next step will take practice.

Write down all those things you loved to do when you were a kid, those activities that put you into the flow now, and what naturally comes easy to you.

Then connect the dots and try to express all those elements into one single, succinct purpose statement that you can easily memorize.

Again, for an illustrative example, my own purpose statement is...

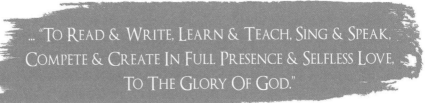

... "To Read & Write, Learn & Teach, Sing & Speak, Compete & Create In Full Presence & Selfless Love, To The Glory Of God."

Before that, it was...

..."To Empower People To Live A More Adventurous, Joyful & Fulfilling Life".

Keep your purpose statement specific, precise, concise, clear, and goal-oriented.

Write it down. It might be two to three paragraphs at first. Then a paragraph. Then a couple of sentences. Then one sentence. Then that same sentence, simplified. Refine it. Edit it. Write it again. Have no guilt about changing it a dozen times if need be. But you must, must, must make it short and easy to memorize so that you can quickly recall it and rely upon it when the bullets of the matrix of life are flying at you and you need to remind yourself of why you are doing what you are doing.

Finally, understand that your purpose statement can change over time as your passions and personality changes. C.S. Lewis, one of my favorite authors of all time, once said *"You are never too old to set another goal or to dream a new dream."* So your purpose statement during this current chapter of the book that is your life may change in a future chapter of your life. That's OK. Don't feel guilty, flaky, or schizophrenic about that. Be open to change and do so by sitting down with your purpose statement on at least a yearly basis—reviewing it, analyzing it, praying over it, meditating upon it, and questioning it to get clarity on whether it still fully aligns with what your soul knows to be true. Run it by friends and family members to get an objective opinion. Do that the first time you write your purpose statement and continue to do it for every future purpose statement you create.

How To Find Your Purpose In Life, Step 5: Love God & love others with your purpose.

Finally, no matter how good your purpose statement is, it will never be truly fulfilling or impactful if it's all about *you.*

If the motivation behind and reason for your purpose statement is to make more money, own a better car, have a nicer home, attract successful people, run faster, get stronger or achieve, achieve, achieve, then you'll never truly be happy, and in the end, your purpose will feel selfish, meaningless, empty, and unfulfilling.

Instead, once you have written your purpose statement sentence, you must go forth and *love others* with your purpose. Bless others selflessly with your purpose. Change the world with your purpose because you love people, not because you want to fulfill Maslow's Hierarchy of Needs or scratch your own back. Follow the Golden Rule with your purpose. Pursue your purpose with zero selfishness and in full love for your fellow human beings, and, trust me, the rewards back to you will naturally come in due time. But the focus of living out your purpose statement should not be on your own happiness, but rather the happiness of others. That's what will, in a way that sneaks up on you without you even knowing it, is what will truly make *you* happy.

Furthermore, don't just love others with your purpose, but also love God with your purpose. After all, you were created as a unique being in the image of God, and one of the greatest things you can do with your purpose is to wake up each morning and, as one of my trusted mentors once told me, *"Do the very best thing that day with whatever God has put on your plate."* By doing your work and living out your purpose each day with supreme excellence, you'll magnify and glorify the mightiest Being this world knows. That's the greatest love and greatest gift you can give back to the Creator who put you here in the first place and bestowed upon you the unique skills, body, and brain you've been blessed with.

One of my favorite preachers, John Piper, puts it this way:

"We are not called to be microscopes. We are called to be telescopes...There is nothing and nobody superior to God. And so the calling of those who love God is to make his greatness begin to look as great as it really is. That's why we exist, why we were saved, as Peter says in 1 Peter 2:9, "You are a chosen race, a royal priesthood, a holy nation, a people for his own possession, that you may proclaim the excellencies of him who called you out of darkness into his marvelous light."

So our whole duty in life, therefore, can be summed up like this: Feel, think, and act in a way that will make God look as great as he really is. Be a telescope for the world of the infinite starry wealth of the glory of God.

Ultimately, live your purpose in full love for others and for the magnification and glory of God. I guarantee the impact of your life will be profound if that's the lens through which you see, and manner with which you live out your purpose.

Summary

Whew!

I realize that's plenty to digest, so I'll stop there.

So now it's simply time to calendar a time with your journal to address these thought exercises:

1. *What did you like to do when you were a kid?*

2. *What puts you "in the zone" now?*

3. *What naturally comes easy to you?*

4. *Summarize your purpose into one single, succinct statement that you can memorize.*

5. *Love God & love others with your purpose.*

Finally, if you're curious or troubled about whether you truly have identified your purpose correctly, then consider these words from my friend Brett McKay from his Art Of Manliness article *"You Know You've Found Your Purpose When..."*:

> *"Your life's purpose — whether as a profession magnifier, human caretaker, faith promulgator, or cause catalyzer — is essential to find, but can be difficult to discern. You know you've found yours when, despite the risk, pain, effort, and mundanity (and no matter the purpose, the mundanity always far outweighs the excitement), you can do naught else but continually return to its trenches."*

Based on all this, I have a challenge for you: spend time over the next day, week, or month identifying, honing, writing, and memorizing your purpose; and then, in a journal, or even better, in addition to that, in a public forum such as social media or at the dinner table with family and friends, write or verbalize your purpose statement for the world to see. Then, as you progress into the next chapter, prepare yourself to discover what the most fulfilling and noble focus of that life's purpose should be based upon.

For resources, references, links and additional reading and listening material for this chapter, visit FitSoulBook.com/Chapter8.

CHAPTER IX

YOU'RE NOT THE HERO

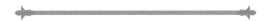

You've probably heard of it.

Even if you haven't heard of it, you've probably witnessed it manifested all around you in nearly every smash Hollywood hit movie from Star Wars to Rocky to Frozen; numerous literary works of popular fiction from The Hobbit to Chronicles of Narnia to the Sorcerer's Stone; and even in Cinderella sports stories such as the underdog NCAA basketball team who claims the crown or the come-from-behind Ironman triathlete who battles injury to take the victory.

In his seminal 1949 book *The Hero With a Thousand Faces*, author Joseph Campbell coined the term "monomyth" to describe it, which is now more widely known as...

... "The Hero's Journey."

Campbell notes, after studying a vast array of mythological stories across different cultures and time periods, the fascinating fact that each of these inspirational tales all follow the same basic story pattern and share eerily similar overarching structures, types of characters, and universal themes.

In other words, human beings spanning the planet across eons of time have been using the same basic story elements to communicate an epic tale with each other for what appears to be the entirety of our human existence.

WHAT IS THE HERO'S JOURNEY?

The basic 12 steps of this so-called Hero's Journey are:

1. *The Ordinary World*

2. *The Call of Adventure*

3. *Refusal of the Call*

4. *Meeting the Mentor*

5. *Crossing the First Threshold*

6. *Tests, Allies, Enemies*

7. *Approach to the Inmost Cave*

8. *The Ordeal*

9. *The Reward*

10. *The Road Back*

11. *Resurrection*

12. *Return with the Elixir*

Surely, for better or worse, you're familiar with at least a few popular Hollywood hits, right? For the sake of a helpful visual example, here is how the Hero's Journey plays out in 6 popular movies:

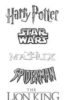

ORDINARY WORLD

Harry Potter lives in the cupboard under the stairs at 4 Privet Drive.

Luke Skywalker lives on a moisture farm on Tatooine.

Thomas Anderson lives a double life as a regular citizen and as Neo, a hacker.

Peter Parker is a nerdy student who is bullied by his classmates.

Simba is heir to the throne in the Pride Lands.

Frodo lives comfortably in the Shire and visits Bilbo.

THE CALL TO ADVENTURE

Gandalf tells Frodo that he must destroy the One Ring.

Scar kills Mufasa and tells Simba to leave the Pride Lands.

A genetically engineered spider bites Peter and wakes up with powers.

Neo receives cryptic messgaes referencing "The Matrix."

R2-D2 gives Luke a message from Leia, asking Obi-Wan Kenobi to help her.

Harry receives a letter to attend Hogwarts.

Harry doesn't believe that he could be a real wizard.

Luke is reluctant to accept Obi-Wan's offer.

Neo talks to Trinity but isn't sure if it's a dream.

Peter uses his powers to win matches at an underground wrestling ring.

Simba, scared and alone, retreats to the desert.

Frodo is reluctant to leave the life he knows.

THE REFUSAL OF THE CALL

Gandalf introduces Frodo to the Fellowship of the Ring.

Timon and Pumbaa introduce Simba to life in the jungle.

Uncle Ben advises Peter that "with great power comes great responsibility."

Morpheus tells Neo to take the red pill or the blue pill.

Obi-Wan gives Luke his father's lightsaber and offers to train him to be a Jedi.

Hagrid takes Harry to Diagon Alley, where Harry purchases his school equipment.

MEETING WITH THE MENTOR

Harry learns about his parents' death at the hands of Lord Voldemort.

Luke accompanies Obi-Wan to Alderaan to deliver the plans for the Death Star to Leia's father.

Neo chooses the red pill and wakes up from The Matrix.

Peter stops uncle Ben's killer and realizes he must use his powers to stop crime.

Simba embraces the "hakuna matata" and lives with Timon and Pumbaa.

The Fellowship set off on their journey to Mount Doom.

TESTS, ALIES, AND ENEMIES

The Fellowship faces Balrog, who drags Gandalf into the pit with it.

Nala finds Simba and the two fall in love.

Peter becomes Spiderman and takes photos for the Daily Bugle.

Morpheus trains Neo to fulfill his role as "The One" who will free humanity.

Han Solo and Chewbacca agree to take Luke and Obi-Wan to Alderaan.

Harry adjusts to life at Hogwarts.

Harry, Ron and Hermione plan to get the Philospher's Stone before Snape.

The Death Star destroys Alderaan; they invade the Death Star and Save Princess LEia.

The Oracle tells Neo that he or Morpheus will die, and Neo has the power to choose who.

The Green Goblin asks Spiderman to join him, but Peter refuses.

Nala asks Simba to return to the Pride Lands and to take the throne from Scar.

Frodo sees the Ring's corruptive power and goes forward alone with Sam.

APPROACH TO THE INNERMOST CAVE

Gollum leads Frodo away from Sam to Shelob's layer, but Sam saves him.

Simba must choose to save his kingdom or keep living his new life.

Norman figures out that Peter is Spiderman and kidnaps Mary Jane.

Neo's group is ambushed by Agents in the Matrix.

The group rescues Leia, but Darth Cader kills Obi-Wan in the process.

Harry, Ron and Hermione overcome the obstacles set up to protect the Stone.

THE ORDEAL

Harry enters the room where the Philosopher's Stone is hidden.

Luke decides to join the Rebels to destroy the Death Star.

Neo blames himself for Morpheus' capture, and reenters the matrix to save him.

Spiderman saves Mary Jane and learns the Green Goblin's identity.

Mufasa's ghost tells Simba he must return to the Pride Lands.

Frodo, corrupted by the Ring's power, no longer wants to destroy it.

THE ROAD BACK

Gollum bites off Frodo's Ring finger and jumps after it to his death.

Simba returns to the Pride Lands and faces Scar.

At Norman's funeral, Harry swears to avenge his father's death.

Before Neo can leave the Matrix again, Agent Smith kills him.

Luke refuses Han Solo's offer to leave, choosing to help overcome the Galactic Empire.

Harry faces Professor Quirrel, who has been hosting Voldemort in his body.

Harry wakes up in the hospital; Dumbledore explains that Harry is protected by his mother's love.

Luke remember's Obi-Wan's advice and uses the Force to help him destroy the Death Star.

Trinity tells Neo that she loves him, so he must be the One; neo revives and kills Agent Smith.

Mary Jane confesses her love for Peter, but he rejects her to keep her from danger.

Simba learns that Scar kille dhis father; Simba throws Scar off the Pride rock.

Sauron is defeated, and Frodo and Sam reunite with the Fellowship.

THE RESURRECTION

Traumatized, Frodo leaves Middle Earth to live in the Grey Havens with the Elves.

Simba accepts Pride Rock and reclaims the throne.

Peter recalls Uncle Ben's words and embraces his role as Spiderman.

Neo makes a call in the Matrix, telling machines that he will free humanity.

Luke wins a medal, and takes his first steps towards becoming a Jedi.

Harry returns to 4 Privet Drive for the summer, happy to belong at Hogwarts.

RETURN WITH THE ELIXIR

Hopefully, that helps you wrap your head around the general idea of what the Hero's Journey actually is. This entire path is best summarized by Joseph Campbell himself when he explains in one single, succinct sentence:

> *"A hero ventures forth from the world of common day into a region of supernatural wonder: fabulous forces are there encountered and a decisive victory is won: the hero comes back from this mysterious adventure with the power to bestow boons on his fellow man."*

I first became familiar with the Hero's Journey while I was writing my first fiction book *The Forest.* To develop the plot sequence for that book, I relied heavily on a book by Christopher Vogler called *The Writer's Journey: Mythic Structure for Writers*, which teaches authors how to weave the Hero's Journey into their books, stories, and screenplays. So I've become quite familiar with the Hero's Journey over the past several years and, as mentioned above, have seen it played out in books and movies, but also in my own life and the lives of those around me...

...the overweight office worker who dares to step outside the ordinary world of the cubicle and sign up for an Ironman triathlon...

...the parents and children who make a decision to venture outside traditional education and begin the journey of homeschooling or unschooling...

...the CEO who pivots and reinvents their business's product offering and mission statement to transform into an entirely different entity...

Ultimately, these are all fantastic examples of people living out what seems to be programmed into our very DNA—the feeling that, as a random Disney princess might say, "There must be more to life than this," or "I'm meant for something greater," and the subsequent decision to venture forth into the unknown to cross a threshold, go to battle, find the elixir, and save ourselves or save others.

Some live this craving for the experience of the Hero's Journey by witnessing it in others, such as by watching their favorite sports team engage in a season of competition, or by engaging with epic movies and works of fiction, or by following a politician, celebrity, or other pop culture icon achieving their own dreams. Others—those who often taste a much greater degree of adventure, excitement, success, fulfillment, and purpose—take a giant, daring step forward and live out the Hero's Journey in their own life.

And while there's nothing inherently bad with living out the Hero's Journey, there can be a dark side to the Hero's Journey.

THE DARK SIDE OF THE HERO'S JOURNEY

Now don't get me wrong: I no way desire to disparage the inspiration, story value and honorable tradition woven into the Hero's Journey. But here's where the Hero's Journey can become dangerous:

1. When we decide that our own version of the Hero's Journey will manifest in some kind of grand salvation of humankind, and we place a lofty and unnecessary burden upon ourselves to live our entire life as a hero, often to the detriment of personal development, family life, sleep, and health as we get caught up in a perpetual cycle of achieving and *doing* rather than learning to be satisfied with the experience of *being* a human *being*. I call this "White Knight Syndrome" or "The Hero's Burden," and have certainly found myself caught in a state of excess stress, a mild guilt complex, and neglect of pressing personal and familial duties because I feel burdened to "help all the hurting people." But the fact is, sometimes it's just as meaningful and glorious to save or be the hero for one person. You can create just as much meaning and impact helping your neighbor weed their garden, calling your mother on the phone or volunteering at a local church or homeless shelter as you can stepping on stage in front of thousands of people to deliver your message of hope or buying a plane ticket to Africa to volunteer in a needy village.

2. When we view ourselves as the Hero of our own story, it can sometimes lead to excess shame or judgment towards others because we, after all, are the champion, the lead star, the primary protagonist, and the principal character of the story of our life. If everyone else is simply there playing a supportive role, it's very tempting and oh-so-easy to fall into a selfish and hubristic pattern of placing yourself on a tall, shiny pedestal while looking down upon others as less of a Hero. This shaming and judgment, which based on David Hawkins' book *Healing & Recovery* is really the lowest vibrational state of human energy in which one can exist, and can be quite a prideful state of existence that ultimately makes those who are around us feel inferior or excessively judged.

Now I'm not saying that there isn't an enormous amount of value in living your life in a sort of Hero's Journey pattern, but you must be highly cognizant of the temptation to place unrealistic expectations upon yourself and/or to judge or shame others who you may not perceive to be as much of a Hero as you. Make sense?

I personally have had to deal quite a bit in my own life with my own personal baggage of being brought up in a home where I was given the impression I was different, I was superior, and I was meant for great things, which, when combined with my natural tendency towards egotism and arrogance, has resulted in me spending many years charging through life with a focus on fame, power, achievement, and "hero status," while looking down upon others who might be thinking smaller or satisfied with less than my own perfectionist, achiever personality thought sufficient. While I have no regrets in life and only gratefulness for the steps that have brought me to where I am now, I certainly feel as though I've spent years of my life stressing myself out with attempts to be enormously impactful, while alienating others because I've viewed myself as the ultimate hero.

Geez. What a burden. And what a chore for others to have to put up with that kind of holier-than-thou mentality coming from me.

But being the *ultimate* Hero who will save the world is not a burden you and I need to carry. See, we don't need to carry the weight of that Hero's burden. Sure, taking dares, making an impact in our careers and personal lives, stepping outside the comfort zone of our ordinary world, and inspiring others with a fantastical tale of slaying the dragons of life can all be noble pursuits; but our identity need not be wrapped up in those pursuits. Frankly, it's not our calling to be the Hero who will save the world. As I told you in Chapter 8 on how to find your purpose in life, our true calling, no matter how big or small our calling and career, is to simply...

...love God (by waking up each day and doing the very best, most excellent job we can with whatever God has placed upon our plate for the day) and love others (selflessly and in full presence do unto others as we would have them do unto us).

At that point, you are enough of a Hero. You can then hand everything off to who I consider to be the true and ultimate Hero. We can, as John Bunyan writes in *The Pilgrim's Progress*, remove our heavy burdens and simply pass them off to that Hero:

> *"Just as Christian came up to the Cross, his burden loosed from off his shoulders, fell from off his back, and began to tumble down the hill, and so it continued to do till it came to the mouth of the sepulchre. There it fell in, and I saw it no more!"*

So who is that ultimate Hero?

THE ULTIMATE EXAMPLE OF
THE HERO'S JOURNEY

The ultimate Hero is Jesus Christ.

Consider this God-man.

From the beginning of time, Jesus existed in the *"Ordinary World"* of heaven, a supernatural realm in which he was no doubt comfortable, honored, worshiped daily by angels, principalities and powers, and sitting at the right hand of the throne of God.

He then, based on God's desire to save his precious humankind and to fulfill prophecies of old, heeded his calling and *crossed a threshold* into our comparatively far more dangerous and broken world, taking on the form of flawed and frail human flesh and being transformed into all the messiness that goes along with that: being a helpless baby dependent on a mother to swaddle him and change his diaper; no doubt fighting sniffles, colds, and flus as he aged; going through the pain and awkwardness of puberty; enduring muscle soreness, aches, pains, cuts, bruises, bee stings, thorns, sunburns; and experiencing every other difficulty of living life on a sinful and imperfect planet.

But that wasn't the only threshold he was to cross, for he not only was called out of his ordinary world and into ours, and did indeed cross that threshold, but the greater threshold for him to cross had yet to come.

While *"Refusal Of The Call"* might be a mildly inaccurate description of Jesus' response to his calling, there is a scene in the Garden of Gethsemane, on the eve of Jesus' crucifixion, during which he prayed for hours, sweating not tears but *blood* and calling out to God because of the resistance of his flesh and the internal struggles within him based on the extreme suffering he knew he was about to encounter. He did not refuse this call per se, but he certainly prayed and begged that he not have to be the one to go to battle as the Hero: *"My Father, if it is possible, may this cup be taken from me..."*

But Jesus then goes on to trust God's will and plan for his life, and finally accepts his quest based on God's will and plan for his life: *"...yet not as I will, but as you will."*

Does he then encounter a *"Mentor or Ally"*? Absolutely: in this case in the form of the supernatural aid of an angel. After Jesus prays for God's will to be done, God sends an angel to strengthen him for the unfair trial and extreme agony that awaited him. Luke 22:42-44 reads: *"Father, if You are willing, take this cup from Me. Yet not My will, but Yours be done. Then an angel from heaven appeared to Him and strengthened Him. And in His anguish, He prayed more earnestly, and His sweat became like drops of blood falling to the ground..."*

Then, after this prayer, came the *"Enemies:"* a throng of Roman soldiers and officials, armed with swords, clubs, and torches and led by Judas Iscariot, seized Jesus, who gave himself up without any resistance (even when Peter attacks one of the enemy, Jesus rebukes Peter and commands him to put down his weapon). More enemies then arise as Jesus is brought before the Sanhedrin and is spat upon and brutally beaten. He is then, bloodied and broken, sent before governor Pontius Pilate, who found no guilty cause against Jesus, and sends him then to king Herod, who has Jesus beaten and mocked *again* before sending him back to Pilate. Bear in mind that Jesus was forced to walk to Herod, approximately two and a half miles, after he had not slept and had already been beaten—then was forced to walk *back* in the same state.

Pilate called together the chief priests, the rulers, and the people, and said to them, *"You brought me this man as one who was inciting the people to rebellion. I have examined him in your presence and have found no basis for your charges against him. Neither has Herod, for he sent him back to us; as you can see, he has done nothing to deserve death. Therefore, I will punish him and then release him."*

But the whole mob of unruly protesters who had gathered to witness this trial shouted, *"Away with this man! Release Barabbas to us!"* (Barabbas was a murderer who had been thrown into prison for an insurrection in the city - and the mob wanted this murderer to have Pontius's mercy, rather than Jesus).

Wanting to release Jesus, Pilate appealed to them again. But they kept shouting, *"Crucify him! Crucify him!"*

For the third time, Pilate spoke to them: *"Why? What crime has this man committed? I have found in him no grounds for the death penalty. Therefore I will have him punished and then release him."*

But with loud shouts, they insistently demanded that he be crucified, and their shouts prevailed. So Pilate decided to grant their demand. He released Barabbas and surrendered Jesus to their will.

Then comes the *"Approach to the Inmost Cave,"* which was an ordeal in and of itself for Jesus that came before the more intense and painful ordeal even began (and is visually detailed in all it's disturbing gore in the film *The Passion Of The Christ*). Pilate commanded for Jesus to be flogged, which was required by Roman law before a crucifixion. For the flogging, Jesus was ordered to stand naked, and the flogging was administered from the shoulders down to the upper legs with a leather whip. Sheep bones were attached to each end of the strip to dig into the flesh more deeply. In the middle of the strips were metal balls positioned to cause deep bruising to the underlying musculature. These whips were designed to tear out chunks of flesh and expose the bone beneath, leaving the skin torn away in long ribbons.

Roman soldiers then placed a crown of thorns on Jesus' head and a robe on his back. The robe helped the blood from the flogging to clot and to prevent so much blood loss that there could be a risk of Jesus prematurely dying or going into acute shock before the actual crucifixion. They then repeatedly struck Jesus on the head to push the thorns from the crown more deeply into his skull and to cause damage to the facial nerves, which would cause intense pain down the face and neck.

After this brutal torture, Jesus was unable to carry the cross to the site of the crucifixion, a hill about a half-mile away called Golgotha, so a man named Simon of Cyrene executed this task in his stead. A whole cross weighed over 300 pounds, while the crossbeam was about 100 pounds, a hefty weight indeed that anyone accustomed to exercises such as farmer's walks or loaded carries knows would be extremely difficult for a half-mile uphill carry, no less in a sleep-deprived, humiliated and beaten state.

Then came the crucifixion. A crucifixion was a bloody, tortuous spectacle and involved a slow, painful death, usually performed in public to dissuade any witnesses from committing similar crimes. It was very gruesome and typically involved being impaled on a stake, or affixed to a tree or upright pole and crossbeam. Crucifixion was invented by the Persians between 300-400 B.C. and is one of the most painful means of punishment ever invented by humankind, usually reserved for slaves, revolutionaries, and the most vile of criminals. Indeed, many cultures across the world associate any kind of hanging from a tree in this manner to be the ultimate curse or form of humiliation one could ever place upon a human being.

The Roman statesman, lawyer and philosopher Cicero described a crucifixion as:

"a most cruel and disgusting punishment"...

...and suggested that *"the very mention of the cross should be far removed not only from a Roman citizen's body, but from his mind, his eyes, his ears."*

He also said: *"It is a crime to bind a Roman citizen; to scourge him is a wickedness; to put him to death is almost parricide. What shall I say of crucifying him? So guilty an action cannot by any possibility be adequately expressed by any name bad enough for it."*

The person being crucified was usually stripped naked. Their legs were broken or shattered with an iron club. Jesus was nailed to the cross while lying down, with the nails driven into his wrists, not his hands, because if they had nailed his hands, the weight of his arms would have caused the nails to rip through the soft flesh and his body to crash back down to the dirt. The enormous nails were seven to nine inches long and would have caused agonizing pain to shoot up both arms due to the severing of the incredibly sensitive median nerve that travels up the arm and into the shoulders.

As the cross was lifted to an upright position, Jesus' full weight would have pulled down on his bleeding wrists, causing his shoulders and elbows to dislocate. His feet were also nailed to the cross, through the top of the feet above the ankle, with the knees flexed at about 90 degrees, which would have caused the weight of his body to push down on the nails, resulting in severe nerve damage to the dorsal arteries of the foot and causing searing pain to spread up both legs.

In this position, a slow and painful suffocation also occurs. This is because normally, to allow for an inhale, the diaphragm must shift downwards, then rise up upon exhale. But in a crucified position, the weight of the body pulls down on the diaphragm, so exhalation becomes nearly impossible, and Jesus would have had to push up against his nailed feet (causing excruciating pain) to so much as exhale. Yet miraculously or as a display of extreme tenacity and perseverance, he still manages to speak at least seven times from the cross, most notably to say in Luke 23:34...

...*"Forgive them!"*

As the difficulty of exhalation continued on a cross, carbon dioxide would have built up in Jesus' blood, causing respiratory acidosis and an intense triggering of a need to breathe, along with an elevated heart rate due to decreased oxygen supply, which would then have caused further damage to tissues and a hypoxic state that caused capillaries to begin leaking fluid from the blood into the tissues. This would have resulted in an accumulation of fluid around the heart (a condition known as "pericardial effusion") and lungs ("pleural effusion"). Eventually, the lungs would collapse, and the heart would have failed from tissue damage (myocardial infarction) and cardiac arrest or even a bursting of the heart (cardiac rupture).

In this manner, Jesus hung on the cross for six hours, from nine in the morning until three in the afternoon on a Friday. After he uttered—or more likely moaned or screamed in a loud voice—his final words *"Father, into thy hands I commend my spirit,"* the Roman soldiers plunged a spear into his side to bleed him out like a dying pig and ensure he was fully dead. In his message *The Horror Of The Crucifixion,* John Piper notes that you probably would have vomited had you witnessed this entire horrific scene.

After he died, Jesus' body was likely beyond recognition. Isaiah 52:14-15 prophesies: *"...he was so disfigured, he no longer looked like a man, his form was so marred he no longer looked human."*

Thus disfigured and marred, Jesus was taken down from the cross and buried in a large tomb carved into a rock. An enormous stone was then rolled over the opening of the tomb.

And that was only the beginning.

THE ORDEAL

See, the ordeal for Jesus had only just begun.

As noted above, Jesus hung on the cross until Friday afternoon. He was resurrected early Sunday morning (Easter Sunday). So what happened during those forty hours after Jesus was buried? I believe this was when the true "Ordeal" occurred, which, in religious literature, is often referred to as "The Harrowing Of Hell."

Allow me to explain. In classical mythology, Hades is an underworld inhabited by departed souls. In Greek the word "Hades" and in Hebrew the word "Sheol" refer to this as the abode or dwelling of the dead—a place of darkness and gloom and the same place described in Virgil's Underworld and Homer's Odyssey. In some ancient

Greek and Hebrew literature, it sometimes seems to represent a neutral place where the dead awaited for the death, burial, and resurrection of Jesus, sometimes refers to a grave and a place where the dead reside, and also to a place where the wicked suffer after death, or as a place of torment for the unrighteous.

In Christian theology, the Harrowing of Hell (translated from Latin as *"the descent of Christ into Hell"*) is considered as the descent of Christ into Hades that occurs between the time of his Crucifixion and his Resurrection, during which he brought salvation to all of the righteous who had died since the beginning of the world. So many consider Hades to indeed be synonymous with Hell, and I suspect this may be the case.

But what exactly happened "down there" in Hell during those forty hours?

In Dante's Inferno, the poet's guide Virgil tells him of how he had personally seen "a powerful one" come to retrieve the Hebrew patriarchs. In the 14th-century poem *"Piers Plowman"* by John Langland, Christ's arrival to Satan's evil underground kingdom is depicted as a sudden explosion of light in a place that had known light only once before, when Lazarus had been summoned back to life by Jesus.

The poem reads:

> "Again the light commanded them to unlock, and Lucifer answered, "Who is this? What lord are you?" Swiftly the light replied: "The king of glory; the Lord of might and main and all manner of virtues; the Lord of power. Dukes of this dim place, undo these gates at once, that Christ may come in, the King of heaven's Son!"

> And with that breath hell broke open, and Belial's bars; in spite of any guard or watchman, the gates opened wide. Patriarchs and prophets, the people in darkness, sang St John's song: 'Behold the Lamb of God!' Lucifer could not look, he was so blinded by light. And those whom Our Lord loved he caught up into his light, and said to Satan:

> "Lo, here is my soul to make amends for all sinful souls, to save those who are worthy. Mine they are, and of me, and so I may the better claim them... I will lead from hence the people whom I loved and who believed in my coming."

In the non-canonical Gospel of Nicodemus, it is described how Jesus, after his crucifixion, descended into Hell and brought salvation to the souls of the dead who were prisoners there. When Jesus arrives, the lord of the underworld Hades bids his servants to bolt and lock the doors, but Jesus shatters the gates, enters, seizes Satan and binds him in iron chains, then raises up Adam, along with all the prophets and the saints, and together, they all depart up out of Hades, and ascend into Paradise.

But do you know what I think?

I think the Harrowing of Hell was an Ordeal that went beyond the description above - an ordeal even more painfully intense for Jesus than the Cross.

The demons, evil spirits, rulers of the underworld, and Satan himself certainly would not have given up their precious prisoners easily. They would not have simply extended their hands and wrists in meek submission to be bound by Jesus when he arrived and blew open the gates of Hell. They would have fought tooth, nail, and claw against this righteous invader who suddenly appeared. I believe Jesus battled for hours against these Spirits, suffering mightily in a fire more hot and intense than you could ever imagine and in a place of such severe and extreme loneliness and disconnection from God the Father that would have been an even more harsh tribulation than any that could be experienced on Earth. I believe that Jesus witnessed, felt deep in his bones, and experienced every last shred of human wickedness, suffering, and shame that had ever been experienced by any living soul and that any living soul would experience for all time.

I believe that he lived the horrors of the Genghis Khan massacres, the Holocaust, the Crusades, the bombing of Hiroshima and Nagasaki, the Rwandan genocides, the Soviet Gulags, every terrorist attack, every World War, every famine, every murder, every beating, every torture, every rape of a man, woman, or child, mountains upon mountains of whitewashed bones, skulls, bloodied shreds of flesh and horror-stricken faces, and every last atrocity, massacre, mass murder, butchery, ethnic cleansing, horrific sin, and last bloody shred of wickedness that humankind has ever committed. Ever.

I believe that he screamed, he suffered, he writhed in pain and agony, and experienced every immoral act of past, present and future in the deepest and painful way beyond anything any of us could ever imagine.

As Isaiah 53:4-6 says:

"Surely he has borne our griefs
and carried our sorrows;
yet we esteemed him stricken,
smitten by God, and afflicted.
But he was pierced for our transgressions;
he was crushed for our iniquities;
upon him was the chastisement that brought us peace,
and with his wounds we are healed.
All we like sheep have gone astray;
we have turned—every one—to his own way;
and the Lord has laid on him
the iniquity of us all."

Indeed, the entire underworld of our existence must have shaken and trembled with the deep, guttural, bone-chilling screams of Jesus as he battled in such a way that the bravest, mightiest warrior among us mere humans could never imagine.

And then?

And then, standing with bloodied sweat, ash-covered skin, and deep battle wounds, surrounded by the bloody carnage and aftermath of humbled and defeated demons, with the backdrop of the black smoke of the decimation of evil, and immersed amongst the echoes of the cries of the thousands of confused and bewildered dark spirits of the underworld...

...Jesus turned to a frustrated, enraged, and shocked Satan, who was now bound in chains and shackles—smiled and said...

"I win."

THE REWARD

With that, Jesus stepped back out through the gates of hell with "the Reward" and returned to his human body of flesh in the tomb.

What was that reward, exactly?

Colossians 2:14–15 makes it clear what happened to the powers of evil through Jesus' death on the cross, defeat of Satan and subsequent resurrection: *"He canceled the record of debt that stood against us with its legal demands. This he set aside, nailing it to the cross. He disarmed the rulers and authorities and put them to open shame, by triumphing over them in him."*

Hebrews 2:14 says that *"...through death He might destroy the one who has the power of death, that is, the Devil..."*

Romans 3:24-26 says that: *"...by the free gift of God's grace all are put right with him through Christ Jesus, who sets them free. God offered him, so that by his blood he should become the means by which people's sins are forgiven through their faith in him. God did this in order to demonstrate that he is righteous. In the past he was patient and overlooked people's sins; but in the present time he deals with their sins, in order to demonstrate his righteousness. In this way God shows that he himself is righteous and that he puts right everyone who believes in Jesus."*

In other words, Jesus liberated humanity from slavery to sin. He paid our sins in full. He gifted us with the Reward of free salvation.

He defeated death to guarantee eternal life and immortality in forever bliss in heaven to anyone who simply believes that it happened and goes forth to live their life's purpose to the excellence of God equipped with that belief.

This means that all the scars that cover you, all the wounds that you may have inflicted upon others, all the pain that you carry, any shame you have experienced, any sin you committed or will ever commit—all of that was completely washed away by the massive, heroic sacrifice of Jesus.

It's that simple. That's the Reward that Jesus claimed for you and I.

The Resurrection

In most versions of the Hero's Journey, the Resurrection occurs after The Road Back. Joseph Campbell describes the Resurrection as:

> *"The Hero faces the Resurrection, his most dangerous meeting with death. This final life-or-death Ordeal shows that the Hero has maintained and can apply all that he has brought back to the Ordinary World. This Ordeal and Resurrection can represent a*

"cleansing" or purification that must occur now that the Hero has emerged from the land of the dead. The Hero is reborn or transformed with the attributes of the Ordinary self in addition to the lessons and insights from the characters he has met along the road. The Resurrection may be a physical Ordeal, or final showdown between the Hero and the Shadow."

The Road Back is described as:

"The Hero must finally recommit to completing the Journey and accept the Road Back to the Ordinary World. A Hero's success in the Special World may make it difficult to return. Like Crossing the Threshold, The Road Back needs an event that will push the Hero through the Threshold, back into the Ordinary World."

Here is where I tend to think the story of Jesus' Hero's Journey strays a bit from Campbell's model - as many versions of the Hero's Journey tend to do. Sometimes there's no hard and fast rule that everything must occur in the exact sequence that Campbell dictates. Sure, the final showdown between Jesus and Satan/the forces of darkness could be categorized as a sort of Resurrection based on Campbell's definition, and The Road Back could be classified as some kind of a journey that happens before then, but that just doesn't seem to make sense. Instead, I think Jesus' journey works best as the Resurrection coming first, and the Road Back coming after.

So in Jesus' Hero's Journey, after he defeats death and claims the final Reward, he is Resurrected in a mighty, triumphant return from the underworld. The Resurrection is less of an Ordeal than it is an astonishing victory. What happened between the harrowing of hell and *how* Jesus came back into flesh inside the tomb? We don't really know what that looked like. It's a deep mystery. At least I'm personally unaware of any record in the Bible or any other non-canonical Scripture of what actually went on "in there" in the tomb or elsewhere or how Jesus traveled back from the underworld and into our world. We do know that the stone covering his tomb—which, based on the size of stones used in Jewish tombs in those days, would have weighed 2000-4000 pounds—is somehow rolled away from the opening of the tomb by a supernatural force. We know there was a violent earthquake that likely signified an extreme disruption of the spiritual forces in our world. We also know that the Roman soldiers, who had been guarding the tomb were found shaking with fear and appeared like "dead men."

There are multiple accounts of this Resurrection in Scripture, including:

Mark 16:1-8: *"When the Sabbath was over, Mary Magdalene, Mary the mother of James, and Salome bought spices so that they might go to anoint Jesus' body. Very early on the first day of the week, just after sunrise, they were on their way to the tomb and they asked each other, "Who will roll the stone away from the entrance of the tomb?" But when they looked up, they saw that the stone, which was very large, had been rolled away. As they entered the tomb, they saw a young man dressed in a white robe sitting on the right side, and they were alarmed. "Don't be alarmed," he said. "You are looking for Jesus the Nazarene, who was crucified. He has risen! He is not here. See the place where they laid him. But go, tell his disciples and Peter, 'He is going ahead of you into Galilee. There you will see him, just as he told you.'" Trembling and bewildered, the women went out and fled from the tomb. They said nothing to anyone, because they were afraid."*

Matthew 28:1-10: *"After the Sabbath, at dawn on the first day of the week, Mary Magdalene and the other Mary went to look at the tomb.*

There was a violent earthquake, for an angel of the Lord came down from heaven and, going to the tomb, rolled back the stone and sat on it. His appearance was like lightning, and his clothes were white as snow. The guards were so afraid of him that they shook and became like dead men. The angel said to the women, "Do not be afraid, for I know that you are looking for Jesus, who was crucified. He is not here; he has risen, just as he said. Come and see the place where he lay. Then go quickly and tell his disciples: 'He has risen from the dead and is going ahead of you into Galilee. There you will see him.' Now I have told you.

So the women hurried away from the tomb, afraid yet filled with joy, and ran to tell his disciples. Suddenly Jesus met them. "Greetings," he said. They came to him, clasped his feet and worshiped him. Then Jesus said to them, "Do not be afraid. Go and tell my brothers to go to Galilee; there they will see me."

Luke 24:1-8: *"On the first day of the week, very early in the morning, the women took the spices they had prepared and went to the tomb. They found the stone rolled away from the tomb, but when they entered, they did not find the body of the Lord Jesus. While they were wondering about this, suddenly two men in clothes that gleamed like lightning stood beside them. In their fright the women bowed down with their faces to the ground, but the men said to them, "Why do you look for the living among the dead? He is not here; he has risen! Remember how he told you, while he was still with you in Galilee: 'The Son of Man must be delivered into the hands of sinful men, be crucified and on the third day be raised again.'"*

John 20:1-13: *"Early on the first day of the week, while it was still dark, Mary Magdalene went to the tomb and saw that the stone had been removed from the entrance. So she came running to Simon Peter and the other disciple, the one Jesus loved, and said, "They have taken the Lord out of the tomb, and we don't know where they have put him!" So Peter and the other disciple started for the tomb. Both were running, but the other disciple outran Peter and reached the tomb first. He bent over and looked in at the strips of linen lying there but did not go in. Then Simon Peter, who was behind him, arrived and went into the tomb. He saw the strips of linen lying there, as well as the burial cloth that had been around Jesus' head. The cloth was folded up by itself, separate from the linen. Finally the other disciple, who had reached the tomb first, also went inside. He saw and believed. (They still did not understand from Scripture that Jesus had to rise from the dead.) Then the disciples went back to their homes, but Mary stood outside the tomb crying. As she wept, she bent over to look into the tomb and saw two angels in white, seated where Jesus' body had been, one at the head and the other at the foot. They asked her, "Woman, why are you crying?" "They have taken my Lord away," she said, "and I don't know where they have put him." At this, she turned around and saw Jesus standing there, but she did not realize that it was Jesus. He asked her, "Woman, why are you crying? Who is it you are looking for?" Thinking he was the gardener, she said, "Sir, if you have carried him away, tell me where you have put him, and I will get him." Jesus said to her, "Mary." She turned toward him and cried out, "Rabboni!" (which means "Teacher"). Jesus said, "Touch me not; for I am not yet ascended to my Father: but go to my brethren, and say unto them, I ascend unto my Father, and your Father; and to my God, and your God." Mary Magdalene went to the disciples with the news: "I have seen the Lord!" And she told them that he had said these things to her."*

THE ROAD BACK

After this victorious Resurrection, Jesus then embarks upon "The Road Back" to his "ordinary world."

According to the New Testament, the "road to Emmaus" appearance of Jesus is one of the early resurrection appearances of Jesus after his crucifixion and the discovery of the empty tomb, and perhaps it's quite fitting for the purposes of the Hero's Journey description that it's a *road*. Here is how that is described in Luke 24:13-35:

"Now that same day two of them were going to a village called Emmaus, about seven miles from Jerusalem. They were talking with each other about everything that had happened. As they talked and discussed these things with each other, Jesus himself came up and walked along with them; but they were kept from recognizing him.

He asked them, "What are you discussing together as you walk along?".

They stood still, their faces downcast. One of them, named Cleopas, asked him, "Are you the only one visiting Jerusalem who does not know the things that have happened there in these days?"

"What things?" he asked.

"About Jesus of Nazareth," they replied. "He was a prophet, powerful in word and deed before God and all the people. The chief priests and our rulers handed him over to be sentenced to death, and they crucified him; but we had hoped that he was the one who was going to redeem Israel. And what is more, it is the third day since all this took place. In addition, some of our women amazed us. They went to the tomb early this morning but didn't find his body. They came and told us that they had seen a vision of angels, who said he was alive. Then some of our companions went to the tomb and found it just as the women had said, but they did not see Jesus."

He said to them, "How foolish you are, and how slow to believe all that the prophets have spoken! Did not the Messiah have to suffer these things and then enter his glory?" And beginning with Moses and all the Prophets, he explained to them what was said in all the Scriptures concerning himself.

As they approached the village to which they were going, Jesus continued on as if he were going farther. But they urged him strongly, "Stay with us, for it is nearly evening; the day is almost over." So he went in to stay with them.

When he was at the table with them, he took bread, gave thanks, broke it and began to give it to them. Then their eyes were opened and they recognized him, and he disappeared from their sight. They asked each other, "Were not our hearts burning within us while he talked with us on the road and opened the Scriptures to us?"

They got up and returned at once to Jerusalem. There they found the Eleven and those with them, assembled together and saying, "It is true! The Lord has risen and has appeared to Simon." Then the two told what had happened on the way, and how Jesus was recognized by them when he broke the bread."

To me, this road to Emmaus story is a quite fitting example of the road back, and reminds me a bit of Tolkien's *The Hobbit*, in which Bilbo Baggins erupts into song as he arrives back to the shir Coming to the top of a rise he sees his home in the distance, and stops and says the following:

"Roads go ever ever on,Over rock and under tree,
By caves where never sun has shone,
By streams that never find the sea;
Over snow by winter sown,
And through the merry flowers of June,
Over grass and over stone,
And under mountains in the moon.
Roads go ever ever on
Under cloud and under star,
Yet feet that wandering have gone
Turn at last to home afar.
Eyes that fire and sword have seen
And horror in the halls of stone
Look at last on meadows green
And trees and hills they long have known."

Jesus' eyes had certainly seen fire and sword and horrors in the halls of stone. He had battled the forces of evil. He had fought and defeated the dragon. Having secured the Reward—the salvation of all humankind—he returned triumphant to a feast. And who knows? Perhaps, like Bilbo Baggins, he hummed his own pleasant tune as he walked down the road away from the tomb, smiling satisfactorily at the scars on his wrists.

THE ELIXIR

Of course, the final step of the Hero's Journey is the "Return with the Elixir."

We've already established what "the Reward" is: salvation for you and salvation for me: all our sins and shame washed away so that our souls are as pure white as snow.

But what is *"the Elixir"*?

The Bible also gives us plenty of revelations about that.

John 16:5-7 says:

> *"...but now I am going to him who sent me. None of you asks me, 'Where are you going?' Rather, you are filled with grief because I have said these things. But very truly I tell you, it is for your good that I am going away. Unless I go away, the Advocate will not come to you; but if I go, I will send him to you."*

The word Advocate here is translated from the Greek word *"Paraclete,"* which is also often translated as Comforter. It is universally considered in Christianity to refer to the Holy Spirit. The pronoun "he" is used because the Holy Spirit is a person. So Jesus said that when He went to be with His heavenly Father, He would send God's Holy Spirit to live in every Christian.

Acts 1:3-11 backs this up as it describes Jesus' ascension into heaven:

> *"After his suffering, he presented himself to them and gave many convincing proofs that he was alive. He appeared to them over a period of forty days and spoke about the kingdom of God. On one occasion, while he was eating with them, he gave them this command: "Do not leave Jerusalem, but wait for the gift my Father promised, which you have heard me speak about. For John baptized with water, but in a few days you will be baptized with the Holy Spirit."*
>
> *Then they gathered around him and asked him, "Lord, are you at this time going to restore the kingdom to Israel?"*
>
> *He said to them: "It is not for you to know the times or dates the*

Father has set by his own authority. But you will receive power when the Holy Spirit comes on you; and you will be my witnesses in Jerusalem, and in all Judea and Samaria, and to the ends of the earth."

After he said this, he was taken up before their very eyes, and a cloud hid him from their sight.

They were looking intently up into the sky as he was going, when suddenly two men dressed in white stood beside them. "Men of Galilee," they said, "why do you stand here looking into the sky? This same Jesus, who has been taken from you into heaven, will come back in the same way you have seen him go into heaven."

The book of Matthew doesn't describe Jesus' ascension, but does contain this definitive final charge to his followers in Matthew 28:16-20:

"Then the eleven disciples went to Galilee, to the mountain where Jesus had told them to go. When they saw him, they worshiped him; but some doubted. Then Jesus came to them and said, "All authority in heaven and on earth has been given to me. Therefore go and make disciples of all nations, baptizing them in the name of the Father and of the Son and of the Holy Spirit, and teaching them to obey everything I have commanded you. And surely I am with you always, to the very end of the age."

So as Jesus returns to his "ordinary world" in heaven, he not only leaves behind the Elixir of the Holy Spirit, but perhaps just as magnificent is that now *his* ordinary world has now become our world—just as it might have been had Tolkien's Bilbo Baggins brought the pleasant, pastoral setting of the Shire to all of Middle Earth or C.S. Lewis' Aslan's Country of blue sky, lush green grass, colorful birds, and beautiful trees had saturated all of Narnia and even passed through the wardrobe into our own world.

Satan is defeated.

Salvation is here.

Jesus created *heaven on earth*. Any of us who believe upon his name are now helping to spread that heaven throughout the Earth while anointed with the comfort, peace, love, and joy of the Elixir for all time.

YOU DON'T NEED TO
SUFFER OR SHAME ANYMORE

God has weaved this entire Hero's Journey of the gospel story into our very DNA.

We all crave to live, experience, and witness a version of this story. Whether we are intimately familiar with the story of Jesus or not, we certainly sense - even subconsciously - that we live in a messed up world (albeit one offered the free gift of salvation to anyone who would take it), that we are broken individuals living in a broken culture, and that we are desperately in need of some kind of greater hope and meaning beyond our ordinary lives: a hero, a resurrection, a reward, and an elixir.

From the beginning of time, Jesus has known of our suffering and our crippling pain, and experienced it himself in an intimate way when he took on flesh and lived the Hero's Journey you've just read about. His response to that pain of our world manifested as an intense act of selfless love: to enter into our oppressive reality, to die a brutal and unjust death, to take the burden of all our sins and shame upon himself, and ultimately to save sinners like you and me with the free gift of salvation.

Because Jesus lived the greatest Hero's Journey that could ever be lived, we also do not need to bear the burden to be a savior of our own lives or of others' lives. He is the Savior already and we need to bear that responsibility.

Neither do we need to cast shame or judgment upon others who we deem to be less of a Hero than ourselves.

Instead, as Jesus so clearly stated before his triumphant return to heaven, *our greatest calling in this life is to simply magnify God's excellence and Jesus' Hero's Journey by doing the very best job we can each day with whatever tasks God has placed upon our plate, then going forth and telling of this great Hero's Journey— through daily action, word, or deed, in full acceptance and selfless love for every fellow human being. If you really want to "help all the hurting people," simply live an extraordinary life to the glorification of God, live your life's purpose as I taught you to in Chapter 8, then shout this greatest Hero's Journey story of all time from the rooftops with every last breath that you have.*

Does this mean that you can't live the Hero's Journey in your own life? After all: it is built into your DNA and a very meaningful part of the experience of the adventure of being a human being.

No! You can certainly live your own Hero's Journey, and be inspired by the Hero's Journey of others. You can enjoy inspirational epic Hero's Journey films and books like *"Star Wars," "The Matrix," "Harry Potter," "Lord Of The Rings,"* and the *"Chronicles of Narnia."* You can witness the inspiring Cinderella rise of sports teams and athletes who defy the odds and become the champions. You can challenge *yourself* to new levels in your own personal life by stepping outside your ordinary world and starting a new business, learning a new instrument, or defying fear and signing up for a triathlon or a Spartan race or a gym challenge or anything else that scares the hell out of you and rips you outside your comfort zone.

But remember: the dark side of the Hero's Journey threatens to set in when you place undue stress on yourself trying to be the ultimate White Knight or savior of all humankind. In the Spanish novel by Miguel de Cervantes, Don Quixote has a similar "complex," in which he believes he needs to do "brave stuff" to prove to others he is important, but there is a certain darkness involved with this Don Quixote Complex that can, in the long run, lead to nervous breakdown, isolation, speculation and so on.

Trust me: I lived with that burden and comlex for years before I finally realized that I could put my trust in Jesus to save people, and my greatest responsibility was to simply tell the great story of Jesus that you have just been told.

Don't get me wrong: I have nothing against missionary work, or helping starving kids in Africa, or volunteering in your local community, or any other activity in which you're "helping all the hurting people." but these strivings must always occur in the context of and with the realization that the ultimate hero is Jesus; and if you're helping those people then the very best thing that you can do while helping them is to share with them the hope that is within you and to tell them the story of the greatest Hero that ever lived.

In addition, as you learned earlier, the dark side of the Hero's Journey also arises when you judge or shame others who you don't perceive to be living their own Hero's Journey as fully or completely or at as epic a level as you think they could be.

SUMMARY

So yes, live your Hero's journey, but with no self-shame or others-shame.

When you structure and live your life in full excellence and love, and people know you are doing that because you love Jesus, love others and have a deep hope within you for eternal bliss and rest in heaven, others will come to know who the true Hero really is, and find the deep hope and peace this bestows upon their own lives; and that's the very greatest gift you can give.

Jesus saved all the hurting people.

All you need to do is *tell* them, and live your own Hero's Journey in full excellence and selfless love.

So cast your burdens on Christ. Then go forth and love others with no judgment.

I pray that you are encouraged by these words, that you unleash any burden of self-judgemental heroism that you may have been carrying upon your back for so many years, you release any feelings of shame towards anyone—because Jesus died for every last one of us—and that you go forth to tell as many people as possible of the hope that now lies within you while living your life's purpose to full excellence and the glory of God in selfless love towards all. You'll need plenty of spiritual "muscles" to do so, and in the next chapter, I'm about to give you all the training tools you need to develop those muscles.

For resources, references, links and additional reading and listening material for this chapter, visit FitSoulBook.com/Chapter9.

CHAPTER X

THE 4 SPIRITUAL DISCIPLINES I PRACTICE (& WHY)

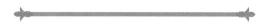

Do you struggle each morning or evening remembering to be grateful for your blessings in life? Have you heard you should have some kind of a journaling practice, but just don't know where to start? Is it difficult for you to find the time to serve and help others? Do you feel as though you're sometimes floundering in life without a clear, defined purpose?

Then keep reading, because today I'm going to share with you the journaling practice I developed in 2019. This practice originated from daily use of a journal called The Christian Gratitude Journal, but my daily gratefulness routine has actually evolved to include not only gratitude, but three additional spiritual disciplines that I've found to be incredibly beneficial for bringing me into greater union with God, with myself, and with my fellow humans.

While there is a physical journal called The Spiritual Disciplines Journal that you can currently purchase at SpiritualDisciplinesJournal.com to incorporate the disciplines you're about to discover, all you'll need for now is a simple blank journal you can devote to these four spiritual disciplines.

In quick summary, each day of the journaling practice I'm about to explain in detail to you begins with a clear call to gratitude, along with identifying one person you can serve or pray for that day. This will help you grow spiritually, systematize a practice of gratefulness, and remind you to take time out of your day to serve others. Each day ends with self-examination and a review of your purpose statement, allowing you to identify what you have done well, what you could have done better, and how connected you are to your life's purpose.

Whether you are simply interested in Christianity and the spiritual disciplines, a brand new Christian, a long-time follower of Christ and spiritual devotee, a Bible study leader, a parent, a student, a child, or anyone else who wants to experience the power of gratitude, service, self-examination, and purpose, you'll find this practice absolutely transformational.

WHY SHOULD YOU KNOW ABOUT THE SPIRITUAL DISCIPLINES?

As an author, speaker, and consultant in the realms of health, fitness, nutrition, and body and brain optimization, I'm perhaps most well-known for my teachings on biohacking, fitness, muscle gain, fat loss, nutrition, supplements, longevity, cognition, and beyond. But for much of my life, I did not focus upon building my spiritual muscles in the same way that I prioritized physical disciplines such as caring for my metabolic health, growing my physical muscles, or tending to the neurons in my brain.

However, after years of pursuing body and brain optimization, I grew to realize that the relatively self-obsessed or carnal pursuits of a lower body fat percentage, finding the perfect diet, climbing your own personal Mount Everest of a triathlon, Spartan race, or CrossFit competition, learning a host of new languages and musical instruments, increasing the health of your blood and biomarkers or "reversing the aging process" are all ultimately unfulfilling, and can often leave one standing at the top of the mountain of physical and mental achievement, yet feeling disappointed and extremely empty inside despite having accomplished what might appear to the world to be lofty and admirable goals.

Most of us inherently know that caring for our soul is important, but we somehow shove it to the side because, let's face it—life gets busy, and it just seems far more practical and immediately useful to go hit the gym rather than sit cross-legged on the floor meditating and praying, spending an extra five minutes in bed in the morning gratitude journaling, or prioritizing relationships during a long and joyful family dinner. Fact is, I personally spent about 20 years of my life, up until I was in my mid-30s, barely tending to my spirit—until I realized that my own unhappiness and constant striving for the next big physical, mental, business, and personal achievement and obstacle to overcome was simply leaving my spirit even more shriveled, shrunken, unfit, and neglected and leaving me unfulfilled, unhappy and unable to fully love others and to make a maximum, purpose-filled impact with my life for God's glory.

Over the past several years—as I have repeatedly witnessed in both myself and others the ultimate unfulfillment of a sole focus upon carnal, fleshly pursuits and as I've observed great thinkers and philosophers while continually seeking for and asking for God's wisdom—I've become increasingly convinced that caring for one's spirit is as important, no, actually far more important, than caring for one's body and brain. After your muscles have atrophied, your skin has sagged, your brain has degraded and accumulated with plaque, your blood vessels have become clogged, and your nerves have become weakened—long after your relentless pursuit of fitness or health or longevity has become a vain effort—your spirit can be just as strong and as bright as ever. Perhaps nowhere is this "soul importance" more eloquently stated than in Matthew 16:26: *"For what profit is it to a man if he gains the whole world, and loses his own soul?"*

Yet sadly, it seems that the spirit is the most oft-neglected component of our human vessels, and that's often due to an ignorance of the spiritual disciplines, or the failure to systematize and prioritize these disciplines into our daily routine.

WHAT ARE THE SPIRITUAL DISCIPLINES?

So what do I mean by the spiritual disciplines?

Spiritual disciplines are specific habits that develop, grow, and strengthen our spirit, that build the muscles of our character, and that train our soul. You can consider them to be the barbells, dumbbells, weight training machines, and running trails of our inner being. In his book *Spiritual Disciplines For The Christian Life,* Donald Whitney succinctly defines the spiritual disciplines as those practices found in Scripture that promote spiritual growth among believers in the gospel of Jesus Christ, and specifically focuses upon Bible intake, prayer, worship, evangelism, serving, stewardship, fasting, silence, solitude, journaling and learning.

Another book that I own, *Spiritual Disciplines Handbook,* by Adele Ahlberg Calhoun, contains seventy-five different spiritual disciplines, including well-known practices such as gratitude, meditation, singing, worship, and relationships, along with more fringe and lesser-known habits such as pilgrimages, retreats, mentoring, centering prayer and care of the earth (incidentally, I spent nearly two years taking my family through Adele's book by visiting, discussing, and implementing a new spiritual discipline once every two weeks!).

Why is a regular practice of the spiritual disciplines so important?

It's quite simple, really: in the same way that mental muscles must be repeatedly challenged to enable your brain to stay young, grow new neurons, and constantly develop and expand—and in the same way that physical muscles must be repeatedly stressed to stay strong, grow new fibers and constantly become more mobile and functional—the spiritual muscles must be consistently trained to be able to experience sustained, productive growth, expansion, and enlightenment. This takes structure, direction, and discipline, which involves more than simply taking a peek at the Bible each morning, saying a quick prayer as you drive your car to work, or ducking into church once a week on Sunday morning.

While these tiny habits aren't bad, per se, they certainly are not going to transform you into a truly disciplined spiritual warrior who can impact others in a deep and meaningful way, into a well-rounded disciple prepared and equipped to defend the hope that is within you, or into a warrior for God who can withstand the fiery darts of the evil one and the constant temptation that knocks upon the door of your heart each day. In other words, the spiritual disciplines keep you from becoming spiritually unfit, spiritually bereft, and spiritually stagnant. Nobody ever became supremely intelligent by reading Curious George books their entire life, nor did anyone ever become supremely fit by hoisting a dumbbell over their head one time each week.

Does this mean that by disciplining ourselves spiritually, we can toil and sweat our way into heaven with good works?

Hardly.

The spiritual disciplines are not a way to earn our way into heaven, but are instead a means by which we are fully able to experience and enjoy the fruits of the Holy Spirit and to fully receive the grace of God that sanctifies and saves us. As Richard J. Foster writes in his excellent book, *Celebration of Discipline:*

> *"The Disciplines allow us to place ourselves before God so that he can transform us...God has ordained the Disciplines of the spiritual*

life as the means by which we place ourselves where he can bless us."

When you begin to implement and systematize the spiritual disciplines into your own life, you'll discover that your entire existence becomes more meaningful and more purposeful. You'll experience a deep and rich satisfaction that outlasts any runner's high or exercise endorphin release you might get from a physical workout. You'll find yourself in a constant, joyful union with God each day, and radiating a distinct peace and hope that others around you sense, feel, and even ask you about.

You are now about to read how to unlock the four powerful spiritual disciplines that I now regularly implement in my own life, and that I'm now blessed to be able to share with you: gratitude, service, self-examination, and purpose. While all the spiritual disciplines are important, these four disciplines are those I've found to be most precious and meaningful for me and my family, and quite appropriate for habitually weaving into one's daily routine: gratitude, service, self-examination, and purpose.

Let's begin with the first spiritual discipline that is a core element of each morning entry in your journal: gratitude.

Daily Spiritual Discipline 1: Gratitude

In studying the writings and teachings of Dr. Robert Emmons, who I consider to be the world's leading authority on gratitude, I've discovered that throughout history, gratitude has been categorized as an emotion, an attitude, a moral virtue, a habit, a personality trait, and a coping response. The word gratitude itself is derived from the Latin root gratia, which means grace, graciousness, or gratefulness, and all derivatives from this Latin root seem to relate to kindness, generosity, gifts, the beauty of giving and receiving, or the feeling you've gotten "something for nothing."

This means that the object of gratitude is other-directed and that gratitude stems from the perception of a positive personal outcome that is neither deserved or earned and due to the actions of another person. According to Emmons, gratitude results from a two-step process: 1) recognizing that one has obtained a positive outcome, and 2) recognizing that there is an external source for this positive outcome.

The benefits of gratitude are impressive indeed. Let's first consider the physical benefits of this powerful spiritual discipline. Research has shown that grateful people experience fewer aches and pains and they also report feeling healthier than other people. Not surprisingly, grateful people are also far more likely to take care of their health. They exercise more often and are more likely to attend regular check-ups with their doctors—not because they are sick, but because they have a greater sense of self-awareness and actually care about their bodies.

Sure, some of this can possibly be attributed to the fact that those who are feeling better physically might tend to be more thankful and happy, but this is not always the case. As a matter of fact, studies have shown that when people actively take the time to list the things they are grateful for, they feel far better mentally and physically than participants of the same health status who haven't done the same. In other words, gratitude's physical benefits are not only correlational but in many cases causal.

Research also shows that when we simply think about what we are grateful for, the parasympathetic, rest-and-digest, calming component of the nervous system is triggered, producing a host of positive benefits for the body, including decreasing stress-associated cortisol levels and increasing oxytocin, **which is a powerful bonding and "feel-good" hormone.**

Studies have also shown that people who are more grateful have better heart health, less inflammation, and healthier heart rhythms, and that gratitude can ward off depression, stress, and anxiety, **which are all associated with increased risk of heart disease.** As a matter of fact, when researchers have performed blood tests for inflammation and plaque buildup in the arteries, they have discovered significantly lower levels among those who had a gratitude practice!

A gratitude practice also helps you sleep better, which has a significant impact on physical health and overall daily function. Multiple studies have shown that those who express gratitude more often sleep better and longer, that writing in a gratitude journal significantly improves sleep quality and that gratitude helps improve quality of sleep and lowers blood pressure.

Gratitude has a significant impact on psychological health too, and reduces not only symptoms of depression, but also a multitude of toxic emotions ranging from envy and resentment to frustration and regret—all while simultaneously increasing levels of overall happiness and life satisfaction! Gratitude also improves mental resilience. For example, research has shown gratitude not only reduces stress, but it also plays a major role in overcoming trauma and post-traumatic stress disorder. This means that being aware of all you have to be thankful for, even during the worst times of your life, fosters an intense resilience that helps you battle stress and get through tough times.

From a psychological standpoint, gratitude can also act as a natural antidepressant. When we take the time to consider what we are grateful for, specific neural circuits are activated that result in increased production of dopamine and serotonin, and these neurotransmitters then travel through neural pathways to the "bliss" center of the brain—similar to the mechanisms of many antidepressants. Gratitude also increases blood flow to an activity in the hypothalamus, the brain section that controls the release of feel-good hormones such as oxytocin, which elicits a positive effect both physically and psychologically.

Fascinatingly, it appears that along with these psychological benefits, gratitude can literally rewire your brain (in a good way). For example, one brain-scanning study demonstrated that even months after a simple, short gratitude writing task, the human brain remains "rewired" to feel extra thankful, with significantly increased activity in the frontal, parietal, and occipital regions of the brain, particularly when a participant gave a gift, or received a gift. Increased sensitivity to other's feelings and emotions was also observed in the pregenual anterior cingulate, a section of the brain involved in both empathy and in predicting the effects of one's own actions on other people. The results from these and other brain-scanning studies suggest that the more practice you can give your brain at feeling and expressing gratitude, the more it actually adapts to this mindset, meaning you can think of your brain as having an actual gratitude "muscle" that can be exercised and strengthened. This also means that the more effort you make to feel gratitude in the present, the more the feeling of gratitude will come to you spontaneously in the future.

These data also help explain another established finding: that gratitude can create a positive feedback loop. In other words, the more thankful you feel, the more likely you are to be empathetic, to understand others, and to act pro-socially toward others, which can then cause them to feel grateful and set up a positive cascade that is highly related to the fact that our emotions and beliefs can affect not only our own mind and body but the mind and body of those around us (a topic addressed quite thoroughly in books such as Bruce Lipton's *Biology Of Belief* or Dawson Church's *Mind To*

Matter).

The Bible also teaches that the expression of gratitude is incredibly important. Colossians 3:17 says, *"And whatever you do in word or deed, do all in the name of the Lord Jesus, giving thanks to God the Father through Him,"* and Ephesians 5:20 says, *"Thanks always for all things to God the Father in the name of our Lord Jesus Christ."* Paul opens his letters to the Romans, Ephesians, Philippians, Colossians, both the Thessalonians, 2 Timothy and Philemon with clear gratitude by thanking God and expressing gratefulness for the churches to which he is writing.

But even when we understand the actual power of gratitude, the deep, primal physical and psychological roots we seem to have tied to this emotion, and even the commandments from the Bible to be thankful in all, it's often too tempting to shove a gratitude practice to the side and instead prioritize rushing, achieving, worrying, complaining, grumbling, and engaging in every other aspect of life that seems to easily distract us from simply stopping to be grateful. I guarantee that the very best antidote for this common resistance to remember to be grateful is a structured gratitude practice in which you are not simply saying "thank you" to the bank teller or supermarket employee, not only breathing a quick prayer of gratefulness over breakfast, and not smiling and waving at someone who allows you to merge ahead of them in traffic—but instead to have a daily spiritual discipline of actually writing down one thing that you are grateful for, each and every day of the year.

This is exactly why very the first question you should answer each day in your journal is based on gratitude:

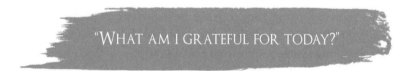

"WHAT AM I GRATEFUL FOR TODAY?"

Here is how I recommend you go about answering this question and beginning your first journal entry. Keep your journal with a pen or pencil right by your bedside so that gratitude is one of your first impulses when you wake. Let this be the first impulse when you wake up. Along with your Bible, let this journal hold a coveted spot on your bedside dresser, just an arm's reach away. Within a few days, the habit will become automatic. To begin your gratitude practice, wake up, take a deep breath, close your eyes, and dwell on a positive experience from the day before, the night before, or even that morning. Do this as you're lying in bed or perhaps sitting in your favorite chair in your bedroom.

As you take a deep breath and close your eyes, ask yourself, "What am I grateful for?" You'll often find it is the simplest of things: the birds you hear outside, the sunlight streaming through the window, the pitter-patter of a child's foot going up or down stairs, the soft skin of your lover in bed next to you, or simply the refreshed feeling of having experienced a solid night's rest. Then, simply write down what it is that first comes to your mind.

Sometimes, things can be a bit more difficult: you don't have a great night of sleep, you wake up with the sniffles, your phone is blowing up with texts, or it's a dark, stormy day outside. This is where the magic of gratefulness takes over because you're suddenly forced to find the silver lining in any situation. For example, two nights ago, I woke up groggy, having gotten just four hours of sleep. The day was cloudy, my wife was out of town with the kids, and I felt less than stellar. But as I took a deep breath and closed my eyes, I realized how grateful I was for the ability to breathe. As I filled my lungs with oxygen, I felt a surge of gratitude for something as simple as being able to take in air through my nose and my mouth. And what did I write down?

"I am grateful for fresh air, the breath of life, and the wonderful complexity of my lungs."

See? It's that easy! Within just a few days, this habit—along with the other three spiritual disciplines you're about to discover—will become automatic.

DAILY SPIRITUAL DISCIPLINE 2: SERVICE

Service is a spiritual discipline that allows you to help others in a spirit of love, sacrifice, empathy, charity, and goodwill for your fellow humans. In his book, *The Spirit of the Disciplines*, Dallas Willard describes service this way:

"In service we engage our goods and strength in the active promotion of the good of others and the causes of God in our world. Here we recall an important distinction. Not every act that may be done as a discipline need be done as a discipline. I will

often be able to serve another simply as an act of love and righteousness, without regard to how it may enhance my abilities to follow Christ ...But I may also serve another to train myself away from arrogance, possessiveness, envy, resentment, or covetousness. In that case, my service is undertaken as a discipline for spiritual life."

This means that, in a way, the practice of service achieves two goals: both helping others, and also enabling us to take our focus off ourselves and the all-too-common positive daily affirmations of *"I'm good, I'm great, I'm wonderful, and gosh-darn-it, people like me!"* and instead move through life in a spirit of unselfishness and a focus upon the Golden Rule: loving our neighbors as ourselves and doing unto others as we would have them do unto us.

In his book, *Celebration of Discipline,* Richard Foster lists activities that fall under the category of the discipline of service, including:

- *Hospitality: showing hospitality to one another without grumbling and cheerfully sharing our home with those who may need a meal or a place to stay.*

- *Listening: loving God by listening to His Word and His still small voice in the silence, and also learning to love others by listening to them with no shame or judgment.*

- *Bearing others' burdens: empathizing with one another's hurts and sufferings, weeping with those who weep, and helping others cast their burden, sorrows, and pain upon Jesus.*

- *Spreading the good news of the Gospel to others: sharing the reason for the love, hope, and joy that is within us so that others can experience the same peace and transformation.*

In Luke 22:27, Jesus said: *"I am among you as the one who serves."* Committing ourselves to serving others in full presence, love, and humility, just as Jesus did—without seeking any reward other than glorifying God—is indeed a lofty discipline worth making a habit in our lives, don't you think?

Consider a few other examples from the myriad of verses within the Bible about service:

Galatians 5:14: *"For all the law is fulfilled in one word, even in this: "You shall love your neighbor as yourself."*

Acts 20:35: *"And remember the words of the Lord Jesus, that He said, 'It is more blessed to give than to receive."*

Matthew 10:42: *"And whoever gives one of these little ones only a cup of cold water in the name of a disciple, assuredly, I say to you, he shall by no means lose his reward."*

This is why, each morning in your journal, in addition to identifying what you are grateful for, you should also answer the following question:

"WHO CAN I PRAY FOR OR SERVE THIS DAY?"

As you ponder the answer to this question each morning, I encourage you to spark your imagination with reflective questions such as:

What can I do to make the world a little brighter today, to use my skills and talents to make a difference? Do I know someone that needs encouragement or support? Is there a way to use my skills and unique gifts to contribute meaningfully to the world in a way that satisfies my life's purpose? What random act of kindness can I do today?

When you set the intention every day to be of service in a clear, specific way, you'll find your self-examination at the end of each day becomes even more meaningful and inspiring. You will feel a deep, rewarding sense of inner peace and joy when you review any selfless accomplishments at the end of the day.

You'll also find that the more you engage in service, the more opportunities for service God will bring your way. You will discover yourself meeting more neighbors, inviting old and new friends over for dinner, volunteering in and connecting more to your local community, engaging in deeper relationships with your loved ones, and approaching your entire day with a refreshing, unselfish attitude.

You may have noticed that this particular question, *"Who can I pray for or serve this day?"* presents you with the option to not only serve others physically but to pray for others too.

Why? There are two reasons. First, when the Lord has placed someone on your heart for you to help, you can certainly take action and do good deeds for that person, but the power of prayer means that you can also pray for that person for a potent "one-two combo" of making a positive impact in the life of someone else and also reaching out to God to bestow His presence upon that person's life. Second, suppose the person who you are inspired to help that day is somewhere across the country or across the world. You may not be able to physically help them mow their lawn or fill their moving van or eat a home-cooked meal—but you can certainly pray for that person! The simple act of praying for someone God has placed upon your heart is certainly an act of service in and of itself.

Here are a few personal examples of how you can reply to this question in your journal:

When I found out that my dear friend Matt who lives two states away was experiencing a tough time in his relationship with his wife, I wrote down: "Matt." It's that simple! Because of that simple note, I was inspired the rest of the day to pray for him.

Another time, I rolled over and looked at my wife lying there next to me. I was not only overwhelmed with a feeling of gratitude about how much she accomplishes for our household and our family, but also overwhelmed with the desire to really "be there for her" that day. So it was her name that I jotted down in my journal, and it was her that I went out of my way to both pray for and serve the rest of the day.

When I realized that our annual church program to feed children at a local poverty-stricken elementary school was kicking off, I wrote down the name of the school principal and said a prayer for him. Later that day I gave him a phone call to see if there was anything I could help with to get the program moving along—all steps I probably would have neglected to take if I had not begun my day with a spirit of service!

As you implement this discipline, service will become a natural part of your life. In the years I spent prior to developing this habit, I noticed a distinct lack of service in my busy, day-to-day routine. Sure, I read my Bible, prayed, had excellent health, took care of my family, and lived what appeared to be a happy and successful life. However, there was a glaring absence of attention to the world's needs for food and water, a lack of humble willingness to go meet and serve my neighbors, and volunteer for charity work in my community. Now that I start every day by listing one person I can pray for or serve, I've grown into a far less selfish and far more aware, selfless, and serving person. As you journal each day, you'll experience the same edifying transformation.

Having established the understanding and importance of beginning each day by refreshing our spirits with both gratitude and service, let's now turn from the morning habit of your spiritual discipline journaling to the evening habits that I recommend.

DAILY SPIRITUAL DISCIPLINE 3: SELF-EXAMINATION

I first became familiar with the daily practice of self-examination when reading a biography of Benjamin Franklin, and later studying his *"Book Of Virtues,"* in which he describes his own journaling system for focusing upon 13 specific daily virtues ranging from patience to honesty to smart spending. As a part of this system, Franklin created his own process of self-examination as a way to cultivate his "passion for virtue" and his focus upon continual moral improvement. In the morning, he would ask himself: "What good shall I do this day?" Then in the evening, he would reflect upon his daily routine by asking himself: "What good have I done today?".

Years later, while bringing my family through Adele Calhoun's *Spiritual Disciplines Handbook,* I became re-familiarized with this evening practice of self-examination, in which Calhoun encourages us to ask questions such as:

- *When today did I have the deepest sense of connection with God, others, and myself? When today did I have the least sense of connection?*

- *What was the most life-giving part of my day? What was the most life-thwarting part of my day?*

- *Where was I aware of living out of the fruit of the Spirit? Where was there an absence of the fruit of the Spirit?*

- *What activity gave me the greatest high? Which one made me feel low?*

It turns out this spiritual discipline of self-examination, also known as the *"Examen,"* can be traced in origin back to the ancient philosophers of Greece and Rome, with one of earliest iterations found in the Golden Verses of Pythagoras, which reads:

"Do not welcome sleep upon your soft eyes before you have reviewed each of the day's deeds three times:

'Where have I transgressed?

What have I accomplished?

What duty have I neglected?'

Beginning from the first one go through them in detail, and then, If you have brought about worthless things, reprimand yourself, but if you have achieved good things, be glad."

Later, the Stoic philosopher Seneca wrote of the Roman philosopher Quintus Sextius:

"This was Sextius's practice: when the day was spent and he had retired to his night's rest, he asked his mind:

Which of your ills did you heal today?

Which vice did you resist?

In what aspect are you better?

Your anger will cease and become more controllable if it knows that every day it must come before a judge . . .

I exercise this jurisdiction daily and plead my case before myself. When the light has been removed and my wife has fallen silent, aware of this habit that's now mine, I examine my entire day and go back over what I've done and said, hiding nothing from myself, passing nothing by."

The Bible also contains many verses that encourage a process of self-examination and laying one's deeds for the day out before God, including 1 Corinthians 11:28: *"But a man must examine himself, and in so doing he is to eat of the bread and drink of the cup.";* Psalm 139:24: *"And see if there be any hurtful way in me, and lead me in the everlasting way.";* Psalm 139:23: *"Search me, O God, and know my heart; try me and know my anxious thoughts.";* Job 13:23: *"How many are my iniquities and sins? Make known to me my rebellion and my sin.";* and Psalm 26:2: *"Examine me, O Lord, and try me; test my mind and my heart."*

This is why each evening, you will follow in the path of Benjamin Franklin, along with these ancient Stoics, philosophers, religious leaders, and Scriptural teachings and answer the following two questions in your journal:

"WHAT GOOD HAVE I DONE TODAY?"
"WHAT COULD I HAVE DONE BETTER TODAY?"

When I first began this evening process of self-examination, I was surprised at the results, and I suspect you will be too. While I often end a day with a general sense of whether the day went poorly or the day went well, until I actually began to examine my thoughts and actions for the day, I found I never really understood why I was peaceful or stressed, joyful or melancholy, and focused or scattered. By beginning to take the time to review everything I did, felt, and experienced for the day, I was able to begin identifying when I was using my time well and when I wasn't, whether I had set up schedules and habits that allowed for deeper union with God and others and whether I hadn't, and what type of practices, mood states and situations or environments allowed me to live out my life's purpose in full presence and selfless love, and which didn't. Each day transformed from a confusing and difficult-to-decode blur to a clear and meaningful twenty-four-hour learning experience.

As you experience the same transformation, you will begin to identify patterns in your daily routine that can be changed for the better, habits that should be kept and habits that should be halted, and even people who drain your energy and people who fill you with peace, love, and joy. You'll discover those things you should have accomplished yet didn't, and those things you may have perhaps wasted your time on that you can avoid in the future. Did you rush mindlessly through each meal with nary a thought of the blessing and wonder of God's creation of food? Did you skip a workout to spend an extra hour at the office, or did you take time for self-care and self-love? Did you spend much of your day in reactive and draining rather than productive and energizing tasks? Was your screen time and consumption inordinately high relative to your productivity and creation? Were you fully present or distracted and absent in your conversations?

When paired with a morning discipline of gratitude and service, and the final spiritual discipline of purpose that you are about to discover, your evening practice of self-examination will be physically, mentally, and spiritually transformative; and, through incremental improvements, will make you a more impactful individual who never ends a day feeling as though you're wasting your time or not living out the full purpose for your life.

DAILY SPIRITUAL DISCIPLINE 4: PURPOSE

The Okinawans refer to purpose as ikigai (translated as "reason for being") and Nicoyans as plan de vida ("reason to live"). Interestingly, these regions are both known as *Blue Zones*, or longevity hotspots with a disproportionately high number of centenarians, or people over the age of 100 years who still live healthy, active, productive, robust, and purposeful lives.

Research has indeed proven that people who know their life and have a clear purpose for which they wake each morning live longer lives. One 11-year long study that investigated the correlation between having a sense of purpose and longevity showed that those who expressed having a clear purpose in life lived longer than those who did not and also stayed immersed in activities and communities that allowed them to be involved in fulfilling that purpose.

I recommend you not only know your purpose in life, but also that you be able to state it in one succinct sentence.

So how exactly does one identify their purpose in life? Simple! Go back and read Chapter 8.

At the end of each day, you should have a special place in your journal to revisit this purpose statement with one final question that pairs perfectly with your practice of self-examination:

For example, if you recall, my own purpose statement is to "To Read & Write, Learn & Teach, Sing & Speak, Compete & Create In Full Presence & Selfless Love, To The Glory Of God." So at the end of a busy day of productive work, time with family, outdoor adventures, or traveling, I might write:

> *"I studied up on what the Bible says about happiness, and began to write an essay on my website that teaches people how to find more joy through connection with God."*

Or:

> *"I taught the person sitting next to me on the airplane how to figure out the type of diet that would work best for them, and stayed present without being distracted by the entertainment screen."*

Or:

> *"I completed my difficult kettlebell workout with discipline, focus, and patience as though my body was a temple of God, stamped with His image."*

You get the idea. As you revisit your purpose statement each evening and identify one situation in which you fully lived that purpose statement, it will become an integral and natural part of your core activities to use your unique skills to make maximum impact for good and for God on this planet with each hour, minute, and second of the day.

SUMMARY

Congratulations. You are now equipped with an understanding of the spiritual disciplines of gratitude, service, self-examination, and purpose, and ready to begin your daily habit of integrating these disciplines within a journaling practice. Be sure that as you move forward into your first morning and evening of journaling that you keep your journal at your bedside with a pen so that it (preferably along with reading your Bible and praying) is the first thing you tend to in the morning, and again in the evening.

When possible, journal in the same place each time, preferably when relaxing in your bed in the morning and evening, or in a chair in your bedroom, or sitting at the kitchen table, or even in a peaceful outdoor setting. You might also find that taking a deep, settling breath when you open your journal is effective to help you relax and find inner stillness and focus. I personally wake each morning, complete my gratitude and service journaling, and say a prayer then go about my morning while listening to a sermon, a devotional or an audio reading of the Bible, then in bed in the evening, read my Bible and complete my self-examination and re-visitation of my purpose statement, followed by another prayer.

As you answer each question, don't feel pressure to write impressively or wax theologically, nor to pressure yourself with a feeling that you must spend inordinate amounts of time journaling. It should only take a few minutes to answer all the questions in your journal (I personally spend about five minutes in the morning and five minutes in the evening completing my own journal entries). Just be truthful, be succinct, and speak from your heart.

Ultimately, I'm overjoyed and, of course, grateful to be able to share my journaling technique with you! Leave me a message at FitSoulBook.com if you implement and benefit from it, and visit SpiritualDisciplinesJournal.com if you need a done-for-you journal that contains the approach you've just discovered. Of course, it is absolutely crucial that, hand-in-hand with a journaling practice, you train daily with the most powerful tool in the universe for building your spiritual muscles: a Bible. The next chapter will teach you how.

For resources, references, links and additional reading and listening material for this chapter, visit FitSoulBook.com/Chapter10.

How to Read the Most Important Book in the World

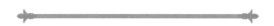

The Bible is the most important book in my own personal library, bar none.

As a matter of fact, I'd say that the Bible is the most important book of all time.

Just think about it.

This book is an eyewitness account of historical events so significant that they literally shaped the entire Western world and a great deal of the Eastern world. A large percentage of people who have ever lived on this planet consider it to not only be a record of several of the most important events ever recorded, but a source of absolute truth and morality upon which families, communities, cities, and countries can be built. The events recorded in the Bible have generated more great works of art than any other book in the history of the world. Because of the Bible, countless hospitals have been built, millions upon millions of humans nourished and clothed, orphanages founded, slaveries ended, and communities healed.

As Daniel P. Buttafuoco points out in his book, *5 Reasons Why the Bible is the Most Important Book You'll Ever Read*, the Bible is one of the most published books in the history of the world, having been printed in nearly every known language and also being named the world's greatest bestseller year after year. Indeed, it was the first book ever used on the printing press and Johannes Gutenberg, who printed the very first Bible, was even voted as the most important man to have ever lived within the past 1,000 years!

Despite being banned or illegal in 52 countries, the Bible is still widely demanded even in those regions of the world where it is a crime to distribute or possess it. For centuries, people have died torturous deaths and lost their freedom for printing, or even attempting to gain access to, the wisdom contained within the Bible.

It is also the most copied book of antiquity. Although the Bible was written over a time period of some 1,500 years and completed approximately 2,000 years ago, none of its contents have ever been found or proven to be inaccurate. Buttafuoco points out that the Bible is:

> "...surpassingly accurate to the smallest details. Its contents, as translated, are as close to the original words of the authors as humanly possible. Only a few words of the entire book (a tiny, insignificant percentage) are in any doubt as to the original words and none of the disputed text affects the message of the book. Additionally, new discoveries of previously unknown ancient manuscripts continue to provide ever greater accuracy to the contents of this book.

> It has been sifted, studied, commentated upon and dissected more than any book in history. Volumes of books have been written about it and if they were stacked on top of one another they would reach to the sky. Where this book can be verified by external events such as archeology, geography, custom, politics, culture, known world history and writings in other ancient texts it has been so verified as to be accurate in all respects. New discoveries always support it, never vice versa. It has never once been proven faulty on single detail or fact, although many have mightily tried and failed."

The Bible contains deep wisdom about God, life, the nature of humankind, and human rational and irrational psychology. It is arguably the book that formed the foundation for the entirety of Western culture. It is described in Jeremiah 23:29 as both a burning fire and a hammer that breaks rocks into pieces, and in other sections of Scripture as a sharp sword. Perhaps most importantly, the Bible contains the most important story of all time, a story woven into the DNA of every human who has ever been birthed—the Hero's Journey of Jesus Christ, which I detail in all its horror, inspiration, and magnificence in Chapter 9.

Should you want even more insight into the historical accuracy and infallibility of the Bible, I highly recommend you read the following books:

- *Encyclopedia of Bible Difficulties* **by Gleason Archer**

- *Fundamentalism and the Word of God"* **by J.I. Packer**

- *The New Testament Documents: Are They Reliable?* **by F.F. Bruce.**

So, if you have even the slightest hunch that the Bible is a book you may want to read, but you have absolutely no clue where to start, or you're already a scholar of the Bible but you seek more direction and clarity on the best approach for immersing yourself in Scripture, then you should probably know how to read the Bible - because - despite this being my own personal approach in the past, reading the Bible comes down to just a bit more than simply cracking the pages open and beginning on the first place your fingers land, which is a bit like walking into a library, closing your eyes, and selecting the first book your nose jams into. You'll certainly get something of value but perhaps not quite as much value as you would have gotten had you been slightly more systematic in your reading approach.

So, because I've personally been immersed in a study of how to read the Bible in the best way possible, I have several tips that I'd like to share with you now.

5 WAYS TO READ THE BIBLE

It turns out that *reading*—which is probably how you'd traditionally think that one would approach the Bible—is just one way to immerse yourself in the wisdom of the Scriptures.

But in fact, there are five ways (including reading) that you can approach the Bible.

1. Hearing The Bible

In Luke 11:28, Jesus says, "Blessed are those who *hear* the word of God and keep it!", Romans 10:17 reads, "So faith comes from hearing, and hearing through the word of Christ.", and 1 Timothy 4:13, "Until I come, devote yourself to the public reading of Scripture, to preaching and to teaching."

Donald Whitney writes in *Spiritual Disciplines for the Christian Life* that *"...most who, like [Johnathan] Edwards, were converted while reading Scripture are also like him in that they often heard the proclamation of God's Word prior to conversion. Faith and the ability to apply faith in every area of life is given to us as we are equipped by the hearing of the Word."*

Sure, one can certainly attend weekly church services to hear the Bible presented from the pulpit, but there are other ways that you can hear the Bible too. For example, the YouVersion Bible app offers a free Bible experience for smartphones and tablets, as well as computers at Bible.com. I keep on the Audible app on my iPhone the complete *Word of Promise Audio Bible,* which is fantastically narrated and is, in my opinion, one of the better audiobook versions of the Bible out there. Some days I will certainly read the Bible, but other days, especially if I'm out on a nature walk, driving, or even doing yoga in the sauna, I'll listen to the Bible. I also think that listening to great hymns, psalms, and spiritual songs that contain words of Scripture is a fabulous way of "hearing" Scripture, and for me, it certainly "counts." You can find one handy music library with sheet music for a host of Psalms and other songs at ChristKirk.com/music-library. Our own family also keeps a Psalms songbook ever-present on the living room coffee table (I'll link to the one we use on the resources page for this chapter), and I'm constantly surprised at how readily I can recite Scripture I've memorized from these songs compared to Scripture that I've merely read.

2. Reading The Bible

In addition to reading and listening to the Bible via our private morning practice and our group morning meditation with the Abide meditation app from Abide.co, my own family gathers before dinner each evening and reads one chapter of the Bible together, usually from Psalms or Proverbs. Later in this chapter, I'll give you several good resources for identifying a structured Bible reading plan that will work for you; but in the meantime, it's important to understand that the Bible itself emphasizes not only the importance of hearing God's word, but also reading it.

Matthew 4:4: *"But he answered, "It is written, "'Man shall not live by bread alone, but by every word that comes from the mouth of God.'""*

Joshua 1:8: *"This Book of the Law shall not depart from your mouth, but you shall meditate on it day and night, so that you may be careful to do according to all that is written in it. For then you will make your way prosperous, and then you will have good success."*

Romans 15:4: *"For whatever was written in former days was written for our instruction, that through endurance and through the encouragement of the Scriptures we might have hope."*

Jesus himself referred many times to the importance of both reading and knowing the Scriptures, and often said "Did you not read...". For example:

Matthew 12:3: *"Have you not read what David did..."*

Matthew 12:5: *"Or have you not read in the law..."*

Matthew 19:4: *"Have you not read, that he which made them..."*

Matthew 21:16: *"Have you never read, out of the mouth of babes..."*

Matthew 21:42: *"Did you never read in the Scriptures, the stone..."*

Matthew 22:31: *"And as for the resurrection of the dead, have you not read what was said to you by God..."*

Finally, in the same way that hearing God's word can include listening to music that contains verses from the Bible, reading God's word can certainly also include singing hymns, Psalms, and spiritual songs that contain verses from the Bible.

3. Studying The Bible

Whitney also says in *Spiritual Disciplines for the Christian Life* that *"...if reading the Bible can be compared to cruising the width of a clear, sparkling lake in a motorboat, studying the Bible is like slowly crossing that same lake in a glass-bottomed boat."* I've personally discovered that my Bible reading practice has become far more "alive" by owning a good study Bible that allows me to delve into the underlying history behind what I'm reading, the origin or root of certain words, character studies, topical studies, and notes on grammar, history, culture, and geography. The depth of my understanding grows by leaps and bounds when I don't just *read* but also *study* what I'm reading, in the same way that you'd be far more intimately familiar with the workings of your automobile if you didn't simply drive it, but also read the user's manual, enrolled in a course on car mechanics, or took apart and put back together your car's engine.

John 5:39 says, *"Search the Scriptures; for in them ye think ye have eternal life: and they are they which testify of me."* Acts 17:11 says, *"Now these Jews were more noble than those in Thessalonica; they received the word with all eagerness, examining the Scriptures daily to see if these things were so,"* and even the Apostle Paul, during his time of imprisonment, asked Timothy in 2 Timothy 4:13 to bring him books and scrolls so that he could continue to study the Scriptures.

Owning a good study Bible is the first key to studying the Bible. The presence of word interpretations, maps, clarity of cultural references, relevant similar portions of Scripture, etc. make finding truth easier than simply using a "plain Jane" style Bible. Now don't get me wrong, no matter how it is delivered, God's Word is mighty and holy, but having a good study Bible makes discovering Scriptural wisdom a far more immersive experience. I personally own The King James Study Bible by Thomas Nelson, and a couple of other excellent study Bibles are the NKJV Study Bible full-color by Thomas Nelson, the NIV Study Bible and the NET Study Bible (which is what I have downloaded to my phone and paired with my YouVersion Bible app). My twin boys own the hardcover KJV Teen Study Bible. You can even get a free study Bible at FreeBibles.biblesforamerica.org.

Of course, once you have a study Bible, you must have a good Bible study plan.

While a spendy Bible study software such as Logos.com is an amazing tool, I'm not convinced you need to get that fancy. There are many other great ways to study Scripture. No matter which plan you choose, be careful not to bite off more than you can chew. Depending on your level of "busyness," if you decide to read through the entire Bible in one year, and you wake up in the morning with thirty minutes of assigned reading to be able to achieve that goal, then you may not have much time left over to meditate, memorize, journal, or pray—so be realistic about your Bible reading plan.

For example, for a long time, I used a small devotional guide called "Our Daily Bread" (ODB.org), which gave me a simple topic-based Bible reading for each day—so I could read for 5-10 minutes, journal for 5-10 minutes, pray for 5-10 minutes, and realistically engage in 15-30 minutes of devotional time each morning or evening. Throughout the year, my family and I are now using shorter topical-based study plans (currently "The Essential Jesus") from YouVersion Bible app, which allows you to either listen or read, depending on what works for you that day. A similar Bible app which is also quite excellent is the Dwell app, which includes music, narration, study plans and much more. From chronological to topical to the "busy life plan," you can find a host of helpful Bible reading plan options on the resources page for this chapter.

4. Memorizing The Bible

There's just something empowering, peace-bestowing, and hope-giving about memorizing words of Scripture and being able to pull them out of your brain and apply them to any situation that life may throw at you. Proverbs 3—one of my favorite passages within the entirety of the Bible, and one of the greatest writings on overall wisdom and longevity I've ever discovered—recommends that we keep God's commands in our hearts, bound around our necks, and written upon the tablet of our hearts, dictating that this will prolong our life many years and bring peace and prosperity. Psalm 119:11 says, *"I have stored up your word in my heart, that I might not sin against you."*

The ability to be able to wield God's word like a mighty sword and as a weapon in your arsenal to fight against anything life throws at you requires that you not only hear, read, and study the Bible, but that you also memorize it.

For example, you will find the Scriptures that you memorize can be uplifting in times of turmoil (e.g. Matthew 6: 26-27 - *"Look at the birds of the air, for they neither sow nor reap nor gather into barns; yet your heavenly Father feeds them. Are you not of more value than they? Which of you by worrying can add one a cubit to his stature?"*)...

...energetic in times you are depressed or sluggish (e.g. Isaiah 40:31 - *"But those who wait on the Lord shall renew their strength; They shall mount up with wings like eagles; They shall run and not be weary; They shall walk and not faint."*)...

...inspiring when you are intimidated (e.g. Philippians 4:13 - *"I can do all things through Christ who strengthens me."*)...

...comforting when you are afraid (e.g. Psalm 23:4 - *"Even though I walk through the valley of the shadow of death, I will fear no evil, for you are with me; your rod and your staff, they comfort me."*)...

...and enabling when you need to defend the hope that is within you (e.g. John 3:16 - *"For God so loved the world that He gave His only begotten Son, that whoever believes in Him should not perish but have everlasting life."*)

So how can you better memorize the truths you find in the Bible? Try the following:

- *Notecards:* Each week, our family memorizes at least one verse from the

Scripture. My wife writes the verse on notecards that we keep in full view in the kitchen, and I also keep the notecards (don't laugh) on my exercise machines such as my treadmill and my stationary bike so I can see them when I'm exercising.

- *Pictures:* My boys like to draw pictures or images that illustrate verses we are memorizing, and sometimes do so on their own separate notecards. For example, Ephesians 6:17 describes "the sword of the Spirit, which is the word of God," so they will draw a sketch of a sword next to a drawing of the Bible to help cement this in their brains.

- *Writing/Journaling:* If you opt not to use notecards, simply keeping a journal handy next to your Bible and writing down the specific verse or verses you want to memorize can be a simple and effective step for memorization.

- *Accountability:* Find someone, such as a family member or friend, who is on board with memorizing the same passages you are, then hold each other accountable each week by reciting the sections you've memorized to each other.

- *Meditation:* Below, you'll learn more about how to meditate upon what you've read, which on its own can be a powerful repetitive technique for committing words and phrases to memory.

- *The Memory Palace Technique:* I'm currently memorizing Romans 8 (which, in addition to Proverbs 3, is one of my favorite passages of all Scripture for life wisdom) and using the Memory Palace Technique to do so. This technique, which I learned from my friend and memory expert Jim Kwik is also known as "the method of loci," and involves a strategy of memory enhancement that uses visualizations of familiar spatial environments in order to enhance the recall of information. Author John O' Keefe explains this method as:

> "...an imaginal technique known to the ancient Greeks and Romans... In this technique the subject memorizes the layout of some building, or the arrangement of shops on a street, or any geographical entity which is composed of a number of discrete loci. When desiring to remember a set of items the subject 'walks' through these loci in their imagination and commits an item to each one by forming an image between the item and any feature of that locus. Retrieval of items is achieved by 'walking' through the loci, allowing the latter to activate the desired items. The efficacy of this technique has been well established, as is the minimal interference

seen with its use."

While it is beyond the scope of this chapter to teach you the step-by-step instructions for learning the Memory Palace Technique, one of the best resources for learning it is **Kwik's book** *Limitless: Upgrade Your Brain, Learn Anything Faster, and Unlock Your Exceptional Life.*

5. Meditating On The Bible

In Joshua 1:8, God tells Joshua, *"Keep this Book of the Law always on your lips; meditate on it day and night, so that you may be careful to do everything written in it. Then you will be prosperous and successful."* Psalms 1 blesses the man who meditates on the law of the Lord both day and night, and later, in Psalm 39:3, David speaks of "musing" upon the word of God, using a word with a rendering quite close to the word for meditation used in Joshua. Author Donald Whitney speaks of meditation as lingering by a fire, describing the mere reading of Scripture as casually strolling by a stove after you've been out for a long winter walk on an icy day. You'll get a quick feeling of warmth, but to truly warm the entire body, you must linger by the stove's heat until it warms your skin, your muscles and your bones.

So you can think of meditation as lingering by the fire of God's word for such a period of time that your body is fully heated by its warmth.

Puritan pastor Thomas Watson comments similarly that *"...the reason we come away so cold from reading the word is because we do not warm ourselves at the fire of meditation."*

Meditation simply involves deep thinking and dwelling upon the wisdom, truth, and spiritual nourishment you receive in your Scripture reading, listening, and studying. Using strategies such as imagination, visualization, mantra repetition, you can, via meditation, equip yourself to become a true student of the Bible—better able to memorize, understand, and benefit from the passage you have heard or read. Meditation on Scripture often involves focusing on one single truth, a few words, or a small section of the Bible verse.

Because your breath is so intimately tied to your stress levels, your focus, and your nervous system, whichever meditation strategy you use, I highly recommend that you pair it with breathwork—particularly using breath patterns such as 4-in-through-the-nose, 8-out-through-the-mouth, alternate nostril breathing, box breathing, and even holotropic breathwork. I introduce you to some of my favorite forms of breathwork that I and my family use in an article I will link to on the resources page for this chapter. When it comes to the spiritual disciplines, breathwork pairs perfectly with meditation in the same way that fasting pairs perfectly with prayer—they are the turkeys and cranberries of spirit nourishment.

As with memorization, there are a variety of strategies you can use to meditate upon God's word, including:

- *Emphasizing different words in the text:*

Re-read a meaningful verse that you have found, but read it a different way each in a sort of mantra. When you do so, stress a different word every time. Take John 11:25, for. example. You can stress the italicized word with each repetitive reading:

I am the resurrection and the life.

I *am* the resurrection and the life.

I am *the* resurrection and the life.

I am the *resurrection* and the life.

I am the resurrection *and* the life.

I am the resurrection and *the* life.

I am the resurrection and the *life.*

- *Visualization or artistic expression:*

Close your eyes and visualize with as many vivid colors, smells, sounds, and details as possible the story or concept you've read. For example, during Jesus's prayer in the Garden of Gethsemane from Luke 22:43–44, you might picture the individual teardrops of blood falling down his cheeks, an eerie whistle of the wind through the darkness of the trees that surrounded him, or even the distant snores of the apostles Peter, James, and John. Bring the passage to life using your imagination, then sit with your breath and dwell upon the scene you have created.

- *Mantra repetition:*

If you finish reading a passage such as John 3:16, you can set a timer (I like the meditation and breath app called Insight Timer) for 10 minutes and simply repeat with each breath the following: "For God so loved the world...For God so loved the world...For God so loved the world." You can even dwell upon a specific word with your mantra, such as "Love...love...love." As you do so, you'll feel the power of a phrase or word sweep over your body as you bathe in the waters of that specific section of Scripture.

- *Listening to a reading:*

I find that with certain inspirational audio readings of Scripture, I can close my eyes and enter into a meditative state as the audio plays. One of my favorite readings for doing so is John Piper's rendering of Romans 8, which I'll include a download link for on the resources webpage for this chapter. You can also simply meditate as you listen to a Bible passage using an app such as YouBible or meditate as you listen to a Scripture-based meditation teaching via an app such as Abide.

- *Prayer:*

Praying your way through a text can enable your mind to be more open to God's illumination of the text and increase your own spiritual perception as you read. You can not only say a prayer before you begin reading that God would open your eyes to the truths that you are about to discover but then, as you read, you can come to God with your thoughts, gratitude, and supplication.

For example, Psalms 23:4-6 says, *"Yea, though I walk through the valley of the shadow of death, I will fear no evil: for thou art with me; thy rod and thy staff they comfort me. Thou preparest a table before me in the presence of mine enemies: thou anointest my head with oil; my cup runneth over. Surely goodness and mercy shall follow me all the days of my life: and I will dwell in the house of the Lord for ever."*

As you read such a passage you may find yourself praying *"Oh God, please be with me through my own valleys, please remove any fear of evil from me and thank you for your shepherding comfort. Thank you that you have blessed me even when I am under stress, and please continue to provide me with your goodness and your mercy all of my life..."*

You'll find that union with God, conversation with God, and dwelling upon God can absolutely make your meditation time even richer with the presence of the Almighty Creator.

These examples merely scratch the surface of ways in which you can meditate on the Bible. There are, in fact, seventeen forms of Bible-based meditation that Donald

Whitney teaches in *"Spiritual Disciplines for the Christian Life."* **Indeed, I have found Donald's book to be an invaluable resource for delving into all the aspects of the** spiritual disciplines that I detail **in Chapter 10, including, quite notably, digesting the nourishment that one can find within the pages of Scripture.**

SUMMARY

In summary, the five ways you can immerse yourself in the most important book of all time are:

- *Hear The Bible*

- *Read The Bible*

- *Study The Bible*

- *Memorize The Bible*

- *Meditate On the Bible*

How about you? Do you read the Bible? If so, what type of Bible reading approach have you found to be best for you? Are you interested in beginning to read the Bible? If so, how do you plan to start? I encourage you to choose a plan from the options I've given you in this chapter, and to begin today. I suspect the fruits that will pour forth in your life and the wisdom that you discover will make this one of the best decisions of your life. Your spiritual armor and spiritual fitness are growing stronger with each chapter that you read and implement, and now is a very special time, because in the next several chapters, you will discover the link between your spiritual fitness and the overall health and fitness of your body and mind, and how to grow all three on your path to a fit soul.

For resources, references, links and additional reading and listening material for this chapter, visit FitSoulBook.com/Chapter11.

CHAPTER XII

PRAYER

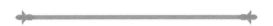

Prayer has been on my mind quite a bit lately.

I suppose my desire to explore prayer and focus more on tapping into the power of prayer in my own life was partially sparked when I was writing Chapter 19 about union with God. In that chapter, I allude to the fact that it is simultaneously breathtaking and humbling to be able to speak daily with a great deity - our Creator.

Since writing that chapter, and discovering the deep meaning and fulfillment I've derived from the daily Scripture reading practice outlined in the previous chapter, while continuing to focus on building my union with God, I've continued to study prayer, pondering such questions as...

...How can I practically implement prayer into my life more often, without it seeming like a formal, dry, or intellectual affair, which it often seems to be for me?

...What happens to my psychology and mood when I pray?

...How did great leaders and inspirational figures from history pray?

I think I've found some pretty good answers to these questions, and so, in this chapter, I want to share those answers about prayer with you.

THE POWER OF PRAYER

Before delving into the practical aspects of how we can and should pray, it's important to understand how powerful prayer really can be. In his thought-provoking book, *The Way of the Heart: Connecting with God Through Prayer, Wisdom, and Silence*, Henri J.M. Nouven writes:

"Prayer is standing in the presence of God with the mind in the heart; that is, at that point of our being where there are no divisions or distinctions and where we are totally one. There God's Spirit dwells and there the great encounter takes place. There, heart speaks to heart, because there we stand before the face of the Lord, all-seeing, with us."

Thomas Merton, a twentieth-century American Trappist monk and social activist, was known as a great thinker, philosopher, and a devout man of God. One of Merton's most notable accomplishments was sharing his views of the transformative experience of what he described as a "mystical union with God." Merton considered prayer to be the most worthy of all activities in which a human can engage, with rewards that are twofold: contact with God, and the attainment of the most elevated expression and highest actualization of one's own self.

I fully agree with Nouven and Merton. There is something very special that happens during prayer—something that goes beyond reading Scripture, meditating, journaling, singing, or any of the other important spiritual disciplines I discuss elsewhere in this book.

Perhaps part of the power of prayer is related to what actually occurs on a biological level when we pray. In the book *Miracles Every Day: The Story of One Physician's Inspiring Faith and the Healing Power of Prayer* you can read about a new field of science and faith study called "neurotheology," which blends the existing fields of biology, neurology, psychology, and theology.

At the University of Pennsylvania, Andrew Newberg, M.D. directs the Center for Spirituality and the Mind, where he has conducted studies of people who meditate or pray for long periods every day over the course of numerous years. Dr. Newberg's research has demonstrated impressive changes as a direct response to prayer in brain structures at the neuronal level. Furthermore, he has found that the longer and more frequently one is engaged in meditation or prayer, the more extensive the changes are in these brain structures.

Specifically, his brain-scan studies have shown that prayer powerfully stimulates the anterior cingulate, the center of the nervous system in which the balance between thought and feeling is sustained. Prayer seems to "exercise" the anterior cingulate by stimulating, strengthening, and enlarging it—while simultaneously decreasing neuronal activity in the limbic system, where emotions such as fear, shame, and anger are processed. Scientists have actually correlated this type of highly stimulated anterior cingulate with a unique kind of personality characterized by enhanced cognitive function and focus, along with increased stress resilience and a heightened ability to be able to withstand and handle physically, mentally, and emotionally difficult scenarios.

The great Thomas Merton, who I mentioned above, described in many of his writings moments of transcendence that he experienced during intense prayer, often characterized by feelings of selflessness and timelessness. Brain-scan studies have demonstrated at a structural level that this actually occurs because, during prayer, activity in the parietal lobe decreases, and one of the results of the decrease in activity in the parietal lobe is—you guessed it—an augmented perception of timelessness and spacelessness, very similar to what one might experience from the use of plant medicine or psychedelics.

These insights from neurotheological studies lend scientific credence and a physiological basis to what prophets, philosophers, and religious advocates have believed for millennia: Prayer seems to, nearly magically, change your life for the better. This appears to partially be because the brain becomes less prone to feeling anger, anxiety, aggression, and fear while simultaneously increasing tendencies towards empathy, compassion, and love. This reminds me a bit of the fascinating biological impact of a daily gratitude practice, which I describe in Chapter 10.

Perhaps this is why many notable religious figures of history who have all who have walked closely with God have also viewed prayer as an integral component in their lives. Many of these figures are described in Richard Foster's book *Prayer* including:

- *Jesus: Jesus frequently slipped away to remote or quiet places to pray and meditate in solitude. In the gospel of Mark we are told, "And in the morning, a great while before day, he rose and went out to a lonely place, and there he prayed" (Mark 1:35).*

- *David: In Psalms 63:1, King David says, "Early will I seek Thee," highlighting the importance of morning prayer, in addition to his vast collection of written prayers throughout the book of Psalms.*

- *The apostles: Although I'm sure the apostles were tempted to invest their energy in many important and necessary tasks, they still gave themselves continually to prayer and the ministry of the word, "But we will give ourselves continually to prayer, and to the ministry of the word." (Acts 6:4).*

- Martin Luther, German professor of theology, priest, author, composer, Augustinian monk, and seminal figure in the Reformation declared, "I have so much business I cannot get on without spending three hours in prayer." He held as a spiritual axiom that "He that has prayed well has studied well."

- English cleric, theologian, and evangelist John Wesley said, "God does nothing but in answer to prayer." He backed up this conviction by devoting two hours daily to a sacred exercise of prayer.

- One quite notable feature of David Brainerd, American missionary to the Native Americans was his praying. His personal journal is chock-full of accounts of prayer, fasting, and meditation, such as "I love to be alone in my cottage, where I can spend much time in prayer." and "I set apart this day for secret fasting and prayer to God."

For these pioneers in the frontiers of faith, prayer was not just a small habit tacked onto the periphery of their lives—rather it was their lives. The following powerful anecdote from Christian evangelist George Muller's Meditating on God's Word is, in my opinion, a wonderful example of what can happen when we do not just read the Bible, but also meditate upon it (as you learned in the previous chapter) and, most importantly, pray:

> "While I was staying at Nailsworth, it pleased the Lord to teach me a truth, irrespective of human instrumentality, as far as I know, the benefit of which I have not lost, though now...more than forty years have since passed away. The point is this: I saw more clearly than ever, that the first great and primary business to which I ought to attend every day was, to have my soul happy in the Lord. The first thing to be concerned about was not, how much I might serve the Lord, how I might glorify the Lord; but how I might get my soul into a happy state, and how my inner man might be nourished. For I might seek to set the truth before the unconverted, I might seek to benefit believers, I might seek to relieve the distressed, I might in other ways seek to behave myself as it becomes a child of God in this world; and yet, not being happy in the Lord, and not being nourished and strengthened in my inner man day by day, all this might not be attended to in a right spirit. Before this time my practice had been, at least for ten years previously, as an habitual thing, to give myself to prayer, after having dressed in the morning.

Now I saw, that the most important thing I had to do was to give myself to the reading of the Word of God and to meditation on it, that thus my heart might be comforted, encouraged, warned, reproved, instructed; and that thus, whilst meditating, my heart might be brought into experiential communion with the Lord. I began therefore, to meditate on the New Testament, from the beginning, early in the morning. The first thing I did, after having asked in a few words the Lord's blessing upon His precious Word, was to begin to meditate on the Word of God; searching, as it were, into every verse, to get blessing out of it; not for the sake of the public ministry of the Word; not for the sake or preaching on what I had meditated upon; but for the sake of obtaining food for my own soul. The result I have found to be almost invariably this, that after a very few minutes my soul has been led to confession, or to thanksgiving, or to intercession, or to supplication; so that though I did not, as it were, give myself to prayer, but to meditation, yet it turned almost immediately more or less into prayer. When thus I have been for awhile making confession, or intercession, or supplication, or have given thanks, I go on to the next words or verse, turning all, as I go on, into prayer for myself or others, as the Word may lead to it; but still continually keeping before me, that food for my own soul is the object of my meditation.

The result of this is, that there is always a good deal of confession, thanksgiving, supplication, or intercession mingled with my meditation, and that my inner man almost invariably is even sensibly nourished and strengthened and that by breakfast time, with rare exceptions, I am in a peaceful if not happy state of heart. Thus also the Lord is pleased to communicate unto me that which, very soon after, I have found to become food for other believers, though it was not for the sake of the public ministry of the Word that I gave myself to meditation, but for the profit of my own inner man. The difference between my former practice and my present one is this. Formerly, when I rose, I began to pray as soon as possible, and generally spent all my time till breakfast in prayer, or almost all the time. At all events I almost invariably began with prayer.... But what was the result? I often spent a quarter of an hour, or half an hour, or even an hour on my knees, before being conscious to myself

*of having derived comfort, encouragement, humbling of soul, etc.;
and often after having suffered much from wandering of mind for
the first ten minutes, or a quarter of an hour, or even half an hour, I
only then began really to pray. I scarcely ever suffer now in this
way.*

*For my heart being nourished by the truth, being brought into
experiential fellowship with God, I speak to my Father, and to my
Friend (vile though I am, and unworthy of it!) about the things that
He has brought before me in His precious Word. It now astonishes
me that I did not sooner see this. In no book did I ever read about it.
No public ministry ever brought the matter before me. No private
intercourse with a brother stirred me up to this matter. And yet
now, since God has taught me this point, it is as plain to me as
anything, that the first thing the child of God has to do morning by
morning is to obtain food for his inner man. As the outward man is
not fit for work for any length of time, except we take food, and as
this is one of the first things we do in the morning, so it should be
with the inner man. We should take food for that, as everyone must
allow. Now what is the food for the inner man: not prayer, but the
Word of God: and here again not the simple reading of the Word of
God, so that it only passes through our minds, just as water runs
through a pipe, but considering what we read, pondering over it,
and applying it to our hearts.... I dwell so particularly on this point
because of the immense spiritual profit and refreshment I am
conscious of having derived from it myself, and I affectionately and
solemnly beseech all my fellow believers to ponder this matter.*

*By the blessing of God I ascribe to this mode the help and strength
which I have had from God to pass in peace through deeper trials in
various ways than I had ever had before; and after having now
above forty years tried this way, I can most fully, in the fear of God,
commend it. How different when the soul is refreshed and made
happy early in the morning, from what is when, without spiritual
preparation, the service, the trials and the temptations of the day
come upon one!"*

Christians are repeatedly encouraged by Jesus to pray. He tells us in the Gospel of
Luke, "How much more will the heavenly Father give the Holy Spirit to those who ask

him (Luke 11:13)." We are to pray so that God can help us to become more like Him in our own spiritual growth. We are to pray for the renewal and the growth of our soul. We are to pray to give thanks to God for all His blessings and provisions. We are to pray to seek forgiveness for our sins. We are to pray to seek help for others as well as ourselves.

Most importantly, we are to pray without ceasing. Here are several of the Scripture references to this concept of constant, incessant prayer:

- *1 Thessalonians 5:17: "Pray without ceasing."*

- *Ephesians 6:18: "Pray in the Spirit at all times and on every occasion."*

- *Matthew 6:5-7: "And when you pray, do not be like the hypocrites, for they love to pray standing in the synagogues and on the street corners to be seen by others. Truly I tell you, they have received their reward in full. But when you pray, go into your room, close the door and pray to your Father, who is unseen. Then your Father, who sees what is done in secret, will reward you. And when you pray, do not keep on babbling like pagans, for they think they will be heard because of their many words.*

- *Luke 11:9: "So I say to you: Ask and it will be given to you; seek and you will find; knock and the door will be opened to you."*

- *Luke 18:1: "Then Jesus told his disciples a parable to show them that they should always pray and not give up."*

- *Colossians 4:2: "Devote yourselves to prayer, being watchful and thankful."*

In other words, our life should ideally be one of constant prayer in which we are continually in union and relationship with God, drawing near to Him from morning to evening. Saint Isaac of Syria, a 7th-century Church of the East Syriac Christian bishop summed it up quite well when he said that "...it is impossible to draw near to God by any means other than unceasing prayer."

The Problem With Prayer

However, I don't know about you, but the prospect of praying all the time seems daunting.

After all, when I was growing up in a Christian church, prayer was usually positioned as a formal activity with a specific structure that required carving out time and forethought to wax poetic to the Creator. Not that there's anything wrong with that approach to prayer per se, but I think that when you consider prayer in that way only, it becomes something very much like the same type of formidable, intimidating activity that keeps many people from regular meditation: feeling as though they need to do it in some kind of perfectly systematized way, X number of times per day for Y minute sitting in Z position—which, as anyone who has taken a few simple and calming mindful breaths while stuck in traffic knows is not necessarily the case. Because of this conundrum, it can be easy to verbally attest to the importance of prayer as foundational to a Godly life, but based on our oft-faulty assumptions about how it should be conducted, prayer often gets crowded out as the calendar fills up with other duties or we simply become too mentally drained or fatigued during the day to conduct a "formal prayer session."

Sure, dedicated time to formal, traditional prayer (or meditation)—in which one goes off to a quiet place, kneels or adopts any other prayerful position, and speaks to God for a significant period of time—is certainly laudable and appropriate, but there can be other ways to pray that allow you to "pray without ceasing" without giving up your job, family time, hobbies, and other activities to move to a pristine Himalayan mountaintop so that you can be a constant and unceasing prayer warrior.

I suppose the best way to describe this problem with trying to pray without ceasing is that we tend to over-intellectualize prayer. As opposed to the simple prayer of early Christian hermits, ascetics, and monks such as the Desert Fathers and Mothers of the early church, intellectualized prayer is the common form of prayer encountered and encouraged in most mainstream churches, paired hand-in-hand with didactic and intellectual sermons, argumentative apologetics, and a focus on "prim-n-proper theology" that can stand in stark contrast to a more charismatic and aesthetic approach to speaking with and worshiping God.

For example, I was always taught that I, similar to the Lord's Prayer, should have a distinct prayer structure in which one opens with worship, thanksgiving and gratitude, then on to petitions, then on forgiveness and repentance, and finally, some kind of official prayer closure. The best way I can describe the feeling I sometimes have with this type of prayer is that it sometimes seems to keep me more in a mindset of praying "in the head" than praying "from the heart."

As I tell my children, it is one thing to know about God, but an entirely different thing to truly know God. The former is more mental, and the latter is more spiritual. Ideally, one has a grasp, understanding, and practice of both. Similarly, it is one thing to pray intellectually, and quite another to pray in a ripped-open, raw, and emotional manner.

Because of this mental, cognitive approach to prayer that is all-too-common for many people, prayer can often feel as though one is talking to God or talking at God in a lonely one-sided monologue...

"...thank you for this..."

"...please give me that..."

"...forgive me for this and that..."

"...whatever your will is in my life..."

"...amen."

In *The Way of the Heart: Connecting with God Through Prayer, Wisdom, and Silence*, Henri J.M. Nouwen alludes to this over-intellectualization of prayer when he says:

> *"For many of us prayer means nothing more than speaking with God. And since it usually seems to be quite a one-sided affair, prayer simply means talking to God. This idea is enough to create great frustrations. If I present a problem, I expect a solution; if I formulate a question, I expect an answer; if I ask for guidance, I expect a response. And when it seems, increasingly, that I am talking into the dark, it is not so strange that I soon begin to suspect that my dialogue with God is in fact a monologue. Then I may begin to ask myself: To whom am I really speaking, God or myself?"*

If you think of prayer as simply speaking at God or jumping through a set of structured hoops, then it may not be long before you abandon prayer altogether, primarily because it can feel so intellectual and one-sided.

In contrast, the phrase "pray without ceasing" that the apostle Paul uses in his letter to the church in Thessalonians literally translates "come to rest." The Greek word for "rest" is hesychia and this kind of hesychastic prayer is associated with a style of prayer now called "contemplative prayer," which is very similar to the ancient form of Christian meditation practiced by the Desert Fathers and Mothers of the early church I alluded to above. Contemplative prayer is simply defined as a wordless, trusting opening of self to the divine presence—essentially moving from a "conversation" with God to "communion" with God.

This type of conversation with God abandons a formulaic approach to prayer. Instead, the main themes that characterize a contemplative prayer from the heart are that it tends to be short and sweet, unceasing, and an all-encompassing trusting and opening prayer that descends from the regions of the mind into the regions of the heart. Nouwen defines this descent like this:

> "When we say to people, 'I will pray for you,' we make a very important commitment. The sad thing is that this remark often remains nothing but a well-meant expression of concern. But when we learn to descend with our mind into our heart, then all those who have become part of our lives are led into the healing presence of God and touched by him in the center of our being. We are speaking here about a mystery for which words are inadequate. It is the mystery that the heart, which is the center of our being, is transformed by God into his own heart, a heart large enough to embrace the entire universe. Through prayer we can carry in our heart all human pain and sorrow, all conflicts and agonies, all torture and war, all hunger, loneliness, and misery, not because of some great psychological or emotional capacity, but because God's heart has become one with ours."

Contemplative prayer often focuses on one word or a simple phrase that is repeated throughout the prayer, or simply at various intervals throughout the day, in a form of near childlike repetition, such as:

"Jesus Christ, have mercy on me..."

or

"Oh God, thank you..."

or

"Lord, I'm so grateful..."

or

"I am here, God..."

I've personally found that a humble repetition of a single word or phrase helps "bring my mind into my heart" more significantly than a lengthy extemporaneous and theologically astute prayer and allows me to, throughout the day, pray without ceasing—without feeling intimidated or overwhelmed by the need to wax fancy or lengthy in my personal prayers. In addition, although I do have a prayer list that I keep for many people I have promised I'll pray for, or people God has placed upon my heart to pray for, I'll often simply draw an image of that person in my mind, or just say that person's name, and trust that God knows exactly what that person needs in the moment. This isn't done out of laziness or haste, but rather out of a desire to be able to simply feel God's presence and speak to God openly throughout the day.

Finally, this type of contemplative prayer lends itself well to meditation and breathwork as well, as I can simply sit still, breathe deeply, allow my heart to fully open, then repeat a name of God, such as "Abba" or "Creator" over and over again, or an attribute of God, such as "love" or "mercy" over and over again.

Do you see what I'm saying here?

It's basically this: Don't feel as though every time you speak with God it must be a formal, intellectual, theological, and perfectly structured prayer. Don't get me wrong: this type of "complex" prayer is something that I think should be a part of one's prayer life, but doesn't need to be the sole means via which one prays. Instead, prayer can also be a simple acknowledgement of God's presence or a very basic mantra or series of mantras that you repeat at various points throughout the day. For me personally, this has allowed a consistent and achievable ability to be able to truly "pray without ceasing."

But there are other prayer tips and techniques I've discovered along my journey too, and so now I'll share the most helpful ones with you below.

How to Pray

Below are five ways that I've found effective for weaving prayer into my daily routine. As you read through these ways to pray, you may find that some particularly resonate with you, and I hope you find them helpful for enabling yourself to pray without ceasing, from the heart.

1. Memorize Certain Prayers That You Can Recite Throughout The Day

Having prayers that you have memorized or written down to recite throughout the day can be one effective way to pray without ceasing. For example, I recently visited my father Gary Greenfield and spent the weekend with him. He practices Orthodox Christianity and has multiple prayer books full of prayers that he has memorized and recites or reads at various points throughout the day.

One such prayer is known as "the Jesus Prayer," which is a short formulaic prayer esteemed and advocated especially within the Eastern Orthodox churches. It goes like this:

"Lord Jesus Christ, Son of God, have mercy on me, a sinner." It is often repeated continually as a part of personal ascetic practice and considered to be part of the hesychastic approach to prayer I mentioned earlier in this article. Often these types of short and simple memorized or ritualistic prayers are structured throughout the day. Below is an example of such an approach:

- *Time: 6:30am and 11:00pm for 20 minutes each time*

- *Begin by lighting a candle, and making three prostrations and then stand quietly to collect yourself in your heart*

- *Trisagion Prayer*

- *One of six Morning or Evening Psalms*

- *Intercessions for the living and the dead*

- *Psalm 51 and confession of our sinfulness*

- *Doxology and the morning or evening prayer*

- *Personal dialogue with God*

- *Jesus prayer - repeat 100 times.*

- *Reflect quietly on the tasks of the day and prepare yourself for the difficulties you might face asking God to help you .*

- *Dismissal prayer*

- *Stop mid-morning, noon, and mid-afternoon to say a simple prayer.*

- *Repeat the Jesus Prayer in your mind whenever you can throughout the day.*

- *Offer a prayer before and after each meal thanking God and asking for His blessing.*

I fully realize that you may have raised an eyebrow at some of the elements above, such as repeating the Jesus Prayer 100 times, and while I fully agree that adherence to this type of rigid, repetitive, or timed prayer structure may not be attainable for many, there are other elements of this schedule that make sense, such as stopping mid-morning, noon, and mid-afternoon to say a simple prayer, or repeating the Jesus prayer in your mind whenever you can throughout the day.

Here's another example: I personally have a memorized prayer that I recite each morning when I jump into my cold pool and swim back and forth. Because the prayer is woven into something I'm already doing anyways each day as part of my routine, it's something that I very seldomly skip, and I've found this approach to actually allow me to systematize the process of speaking to God each morning:

"Our Father in heaven, I surrender all to you

Turn me into the father and husband you would have for me to be

Into a man who will fulfill your great commission

And remove from me all judgment of others

Grant me your heavenly wisdom

Remove from me my worldly temptations

Teach me to listen to your still, small voice in the silence

And fill me with your peace, your love, and your joy. Amen."

Of course, another example of a prayer that you can memorize and recite from your heart throughout the day is the Lord's Prayer, from Matthew 6:6-13 in the Bible:

"Our Father which art in heaven,

Hallowed be Thy name.

Thy kingdom come.

Thy will be done in earth,

as it is in heaven.

Give us this day our daily bread.

And forgive us our debts,

as we forgive our debtors.

And lead us not into temptation,

but deliver us from evil:

For Thine is the kingdom, and the power,

and the glory, for ever.

Amen."

2. Keep A Prayer List

In the previous chapter, I filled you in on an app that my entire family uses called YouBible. In addition to offering the convenience of a host of done-for-you Bible reading plans, it also includes a handy prayer list that you can share with anyone else who is your friend or follower on the YouBible app (or you can just keep the prayer list to yourself if you'd like). Since I'm prone to forget people I've offered to pray for or specific things I want to pray about it, I find it tremendously helpful to be able to simply open the prayer list on my phone, tablet or computer and have an at-a-glance list of anything or anyone that I want to bring before God. Each morning and evening, my family gathers together for our meditation and journaling practice, and as part of that, use the prayer list to remind us what to pray about. I know others who keep a prayer journal by their bedside or even on a scrap of paper tucked away into their Bible.

Some people find that an ever-expanding prayer list like this can be intimidating and lead to similar daunting or time-consuming issues with prayer that I've described earlier in this article, but here's the thing: you don't have to go through the *entire list* every time you pray. Often, I'll spend an entire day in multiple prayer sessions attending to just a few people or items who are on the list. What's most important is to actually have a written log *somewhere* of, for example, people who you've told you would pray for, along with the details of what you're praying about for them. Consider this to be built-in accountability for your prayer practice.

3. Pray Regularly With A Spouse Or Loved One

One of the best pieces of marriage advice that I ever received was to pray with my wife each night before bed. Although I've slightly adapted that advice to now instead pray with the entire family every night before bed (usually gathered in my twin boys' room) the concept remains the same as that outlined in Matthew 18:20: *"For where two or three gather in my name, there am I with them."* Not only does the power of prayer seem to become even more magnified when someone is there praying with you, muttering *"Amens"* and *"Yes, Lords"* and squeezing your shoulder or your hand as you pray, but, similar to a prayer list, having someone with which you regularly pray builds in accountability and encouragement to your practice of prayer.

However, it's important that there be an understanding between you and whoever it is you're praying with. It can't be a loosy-goosy, sometimes-remember/sometimes-don't morning or evening prayer routine. It needs to be as automatic as brushing your teeth, or pulling on your pajamas or flipping off the lights: whether it's a family affair or a spousal relationship, there must be a dedicated, identifiable time or times that you all pray together. For the Greenfield family, regular prayer times together as a family come at least three times per day: after morning meditation, before dinner, and before bed. I would encourage you to engage as many of your family members or loved ones as possible to join you in a practice of prayer, and to also, if possible, share the same prayer list.

4. Combine Fasting And Prayer

Jesus experienced an extraordinary transformation following his forty-day stint of fasting in a rugged mountain wilderness location near the Jordan River.

It was only after this experience that Jesus returned to Galilee an entirely new man and commenced to perform a host of impressive miracles. It turns out that the combination of prayer and fasting has deep historical roots in Christianity. In the Old Testament, fasting combined with prayer was used when there was a deep need and dependence for God's work in one's life or in a particular set of often dire circumstances, such as abject helplessness in the face of actual or anticipated calamity. Prayer and fasting are historically combined for periods of mourning, repentance or deep spiritual need.

For example, Daniel 9:3 says, *"So I turned to the Lord God and pleaded with him in prayer and petition, in fasting, and in sackcloth and ashes."* King David prayed and fasted over his sick child in 2 Samuel 12:16, and wept before the Lord in his fasted state in earnest intercession in verses 21 and 22 of that same chapter. In Esther 4:16, Esther urges Mordecai and the Jews to fast for her before she planned to appear before her husband the king. The first chapter of Nehemiah describes Nehemiah combining prayer and fasting because of his deep distress over the distressing news that Jerusalem had been desolated. We are told in Luke 2:37 that the prophetess Anna *"never left the temple but worshiped night and day, fasting and praying"*.

The probable reason that fasting and prayer can be so powerful is that fasting dramatically sharpens the mind, reduces distractions or sluggishness brought on by calorie consumption, and denies the body in a manner that strengthens the resilience of soul and spirit, often causing prayers to become more deep, thoughtful and meaningful. In the book *Atomic Power With God* (which I recommend you read as an excellent, classic treatise on how to combine prayer and fasting), author Franklin Hall describes prayer and fasting as follows:

"PRAYER and FASTING move the hand that controls the Universe. When a person shuts out the world for a season of prayer, fasting, and consecration, it opens the heart of God and the windows of heaven and brings the forces of God into action on your behalf. When a person begins to fast and pray, they become a channel for the Holy Ghost to flow through as a yielded vessel. Fasting without much prayer is like having a car with no gas to operate the vehicle. Your set-aside season of fasting should be accompanied by much

more prayer than just your normal daily prayer life of one hour a day. After about the third day of your fast, the flesh barrier has basically been broken through and these first few days of crucifying the flesh can feel like you are accomplishing nothing—because most of the time you FEEL nothing. Now, there are those special times when you are able to weep and cry under the power of God during these first few days of fasting, but my experience has been that it's very rare. Remember ... fasting without prayer is only a diet. You MUST find a secret place and spend time with HIM alone while you fast. You need to find a place where you can speak things in private and take authority over personal circumstances you are addressing without feeling intimidated or feel like someone else is listening."

While I don't necessarily think that to be spiritually fit you must be in a state of constant fasting and prayer, I do encourage you, when there is a particularly problematic, distressing or meaningful thing that you need to pray about, that you consider a day of fasting, and that you take the twenty minutes to an hour that you'd normally spend eating a breakfast, lunch or dinner on that day to instead slip away for a deeper state of meditation and prayer than you would normally otherwise be able to experience.

5. Regularly Ask Others "How can I pray for you?"

I've been making it a habit, when I finish a dinner party, a social gathering, a phone conversation or any other meeting with a friend or friends, to ask around the table or to a specific person one simple question...

..."How can I pray for you?"

I'm constantly amazed at how open, transparent, honest and vulnerable the replies can be, even from those who would not classify themselves as spiritual or religious, but who nonetheless seem quite open to being prayed for. Often, someone will share a health condition, a personal struggle, a business or relationship difficulty, a need for clarity, insight, wisdom or discernment, or some other trouble, worry or setback that they hadn't brought up at any other point in the conversation. Often, I'll pray with them right then and there, but other times I will, as an alternative to or in addition to that, jot that person and their specific need down in the prayer list I alluded to earlier so that their need stays top of mind in my prayer sessions for that week. If you adopt this practice, I encourage you to text, call or speak with that person one to two weeks afterwards to check in and see how they are doing with the particular issue you've been praying for them about. This can often lead to even more meaningful discussion and, for those who may not know or understand God, faith or salvation, the opportunity to open their eyes to love and light of salvation and hope that is within you.

Summary

So there you have it: prayer is powerful, but it can be tricky sometimes to weave it into your day, especially if you "overthink" or excessively intellectualize it. But approaching prayer from a more pure and simple, near-childlike perspective of openly speaking to God throughout the day in a form of contemplative prayer - even with single words, phrases or mantras - you can indeed "pray without ceasing", without necessarily spending the entire day on your knees in your bedroom.

In addition, memorizing certain prayers, keeping a prayer list, praying regularly with a loved one, combining fasting and prayer, and regularly asking others how you can pray for them can be incredibly helpful for building prayer into your life in a meaningful and profound way that, as you've just learned, can literally change your biology and neurology for the better while simultaneously bringing you closer to daily union with God.

Finally, I've found the following three books to be incredible resources for learning more about prayer, and well worth a read:

* *Spiritual Disciplines for the Christian Life* by Donald S. Whitney

* *The Celebration of Discipline* by Richard Foster

* *Prayer* by Richard Foster (particularly good for learning different prayers for different occasions, such as contemplation, healing, blessing, forgiveness, and rest).

How about you? How do you think about prayer? Do you have favorite prayers that you rely upon on a regular basis? Do you find that certain forms of prayer bring you closer to union with God? Have you discovered resources, handbooks, journals, or other literary tools or apps you use to support a prayer practice? I encourage you to hunt down and weave as many prayer-enhancing tools and tactics into your life as possible. Your spiritual armor and spiritual fitness are growing stronger with each chapter that you read and implement, and now in the next several chapters, you will discover the link between this spiritual fitness and the overall health and fitness of your body and mind, and how to grow all three on your path to a fit soul.

For resources, references, links and additional reading and listening material for this chapter, visit FitSoulBook.com/Chapter12.

BREATHTAKING

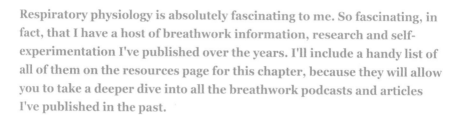

Respiratory physiology is absolutely fascinating to me. So fascinating, in fact, that I have a host of breathwork information, research and self-experimentation I've published over the years. I'll include a handy list of all of them on the resources page for this chapter, because they will allow you to take a deeper dive into all the breathwork podcasts and articles I've published in the past.

Just pause for a moment, take a deep breath in through your nose, then out through your mouth, releasing all tension in your body as you do so, and then dwell upon the complex and wonderful science of that single breath.

That single breath you just took began with your nose. Your nasal passages are quite similar to a high-tech air conditioning and purifying system. They filter out large dust particles and microbial spores via the mucous membrane that lines your nasal cavity, where sticky mucus is secreted to trap and dispose of impurities. The nasal passages warm and humidify the air you breathe, primarily by the means of a rich blood supply below the mucous membrane. This blood acts as a kind of chemical cleanser of your respiration. Despite a microsecond contact time with the nasal mucosa, your inspired air during this time is cleared of ozone, sulfur dioxide, and other water-soluble pollutant gases (far better than it is cleared by breathing through your mouth, in fact).

Nitric oxide, or NO, is a very important substance produced in large quantities in the nasal sinuses. When you inhale through your nose, NO accompanies the inhaled air in order to dilate the bronchial tubes to allow the air to pass through easily. NO also has antimicrobial properties that can kill viruses and bacteria that have escaped from the cilia inside your nose and throat (interestingly, including problematic compounds such as the coronavirus). NO also causes the blood vessels inside your lungs to dilate, which allows oxygen to be transferred to your blood more easily (this phenomenon also does not occur when you breathe through your mouth).

After being warmed and cleaned, the air passes into your windpipe (trachea) and from there it diverts into two large branches—the main bronchi (where it continues the cleaning process via removal of finer particles), followed by progressive branching into increasingly smaller bronchi called bronchioli. The mucous membrane lining these bronchi also contains cells with cilia, which are tiny whip-like hairs that beat directionally to move a layer of mucus upwards toward your throat, where the mucus and the particles it has entrapped can be swallowed.

Each bronchiolus terminates in a tiny air sac called an alveolus, which contain enzymes to dissolve mucus, thus keeping the alveoli from getting "plugged up" by mucus, along with a soapy substance called surfactant, which keeps the moist alveoli from collapsing due to surface tension. Within the walls of each these 800 million-ish alveolus in your lungs are tiny, tightly packed blood vessels, or capillaries, with incredibly thin walls where gas exchange can take place. Used, deoxygenated blood coming into your lungs from the veins via your heart contains a surplus of carbon dioxide, which is then exchanged for oxygen through the alveoli. The prepared, oxygenated blood is then returned to your heart for circulation to the rest of your body—where the oxygen then drives all the metabolic reactions that give your cells life. This entire sequence only takes approximately 1.5 seconds, and during that process, your heart is spreading 8 tons of blood over a lung area of half the size of a tennis court, then shunting it back into circulation...about 100,000 times a day!

This incredible respiratory system I've just described has such an abundance of functional reserve built into it that studies have shown people can lose nearly ¾ of their lung tissue before serious respiratory difficulty develops! It is a staggeringly elegant system, showing every sign of being a complex, intelligently designed loop that allows you to maintain energy and life via something as seemingly simple as your breath.

5 Ways A Breathwork Practice Can Make Your Life Better

But breathing goes far beyond a mere exchange of oxygen and carbon dioxide.

For example, in the fascinating book *"Breathing as Spiritual Practice: Experiencing the Presence of God,"* author Will Johnson describes how Western spiritual traditions, such as the Book of Genesis, the Jewish teachings of Ruach, and the poetry of Rumi, all contain "hidden" instructions for meditative breathing practices. He explains how breathing practices can bring you closer to a direct experience of the palpable presence of God. I've personally found many of his ideas to be quite insightful, and have been able to positively enhance my long walks, spiritual disciplines, meditation practice, connection to God, prayer time, sexual experiences, stress response, and much more—simply by using my breath.

Here are five such examples...

First, your breath is crucial for full mindfulness and *presence*.

It's absolutely mind-boggling the extreme clarity that one simple, focused breath can give you—and earth-shattering what can occur in your brain with 5, 10, 20, 30, or even 60 minutes of breathwork. But start small. Any time you desire to be more present and mindful—whether you are playing with a child, sitting in traffic, firing through emails, preparing for a workout, getting ready to eat a meal, or reading a meaningful text—simply take one to three slow, mindful breaths.

The basic technique for mindful breathing is to focus your attention on your breath (the inhale and exhale) with openness and childlike curiosity. As you inhale (preferably through the nose) and exhale (preferably through slightly pursed lips), even if it is just for sixty seconds, you should:

- Notice how your body feels.

- Bring your awareness to any part of your body that feels tense, then contract and subsequently relax those muscles.

- Next, bring your awareness back to your breath.

- Notice where you feel the breath most in your body.

- Settle into relaxation as you follow the sensation of each inhale and exhale.

- If your mind wanders, simply acknowledge the sensations, thoughts or feelings that arise with open curiosity, like wispy clouds passing from one ear across to the other ear, and then let them go.

- Continue to gently direct your attention back to your breath for as long you'd like.

I suspect that the reason this type of "pause" allows you to be present and mindful is that the relaxed breathing activates your restful parasympathetic nervous system, shifting you from a state of hyperalertness, scanning for danger, and somewhat shallow focus to a more blissful state of depth and awareness towards whichever activity you are engaged in. Of course, this tactic can be used in reverse also: you can do one to three minutes of rapid "hyperventilation" breathing to psyche you up for a workout, wake you up in the morning, or prepare you for a competition. Breath is in fact the best free method you own to shift your nervous system in any direction you desire. Learn that skill, and your life will be better for it. In my article, "How To Blast You (And Your Child's!) Physical, Mental, & Spiritual Resilience Through The Roof With Breathwork," I give you plenty of tools and tactics to do so, and I'll link to that article on the resources page for this chapter.

Second, your breath can optimize your *sleep.*

While there is a multitude of forms of relaxing breathwork to prepare for sleep, several of which I discuss in Chapter 16 and also in Chapter 3 of my book *Boundless,* two of my favorite forms of nighttime breathing are a "double-inhale-to-exhale" and a "4-7-8" pattern. For the former, my friend and brilliant neuroscientist, Dr. Andrew Huberman, claims that breaking up one long inhale as a double inhale through your nose and then exhaling through your mouth can calm you instantly. It definitely seems to work. In addition, Dr. Andrew Weil, in a podcast interview with me, described how he favors the 4-7-8 protocol, and this pattern of a "4 count in-7 count hold-8 count out" also seems to work quite well, probably because, based on a concept called "cardiac coherence," a long, relaxed exhale activates the parasympathetic nervous system, slows the heart rate, and increases the heart rate variability—a sign of overall nervous system resilience and a de-stressed state (notably, I have found a 4-8 pattern with just a brief pause at the top of the inhale to work just as well as a 4-7-8 pattern).

But I think the benefits of a long, relaxed exhale go beyond the nervous system. As I mention in Chapter 16, I also view this long breath out as a sign of trust in God—a trust that the next breath in will be there waiting to fill me with life. So each night, as I fall asleep to the gentle diaphragmatic lull of my own "4-count-in-8-count-out" breathwork pattern, I'm silently thanking God and trusting God that there will be yet more oxygen available for me for my next inhale. Indeed, the mere act of mindful breathing combined with a silent gratefulness to God for each and every breath is a wonderful practice, and one I recommend you try the next time you're stuck in twenty minutes of traffic. After all, our great Creator smiles when we worship Him, and I certainly think that no king would complain of a subject entering their throne room for several minutes and saying with the deepest gratitude with each breath..."*Thank you...thank you...thank you...*"

The opposite also holds true. Hastily sucking your breath in with shallow chest breathing and rapid exhales is not only a fast track to activating your fight-and-flight sympathetic nervous system, but also a sign that you've set aside trust in God to instead greedily consume the air around you like a glutton stuffing their face to sickness with every morsel they can find at the dinner table, because who knows if they'll be blessed with the same provisions the next day?

Third, certain breathing strategies can vastly enhance your sexual experience.

In *Finding God Through Sex* spiritual sexuality author David Deida presents a way to make love in which sex becomes an erotic act of devotional surrender that he describes as "making love, magnifying love, from the boundless depth of your heart through every inch of your body and in merger with your lover." As you can also read in David's book *Way Of The Superior Man,* breath is an integral part of the practice that David teaches. Breathwork paired with sex has absolutely transformed my own lovemaking experience in such a powerful way that I often wish (with no regrets, but only gratefulness) that I'd discovered it earlier!

During sex, conscious breathing can help connect you with your body and intensify your sensations. In fact, breathing may be the most underused tool in your sexual "arsenal." With the right type of breathing during sex, you can awaken sensitive nerve endings and experiment with different rhythms, patterns, and even shifts in body temperatures and blood or "chi" flow.

For example, during foreplay, you can simply rock back and forth with your partner, your face close to theirs, timing your breath so that as your partner exhales, you inhale, and vice versa. Play with your breath this way as you face each other—rubbing noses together, brushing cheeks together, teasing but not kissing, gently touching lips occasionally, and continuing to breathe together for several minutes. During this time, you can breathe onto a sensitive part of your partner's body to warm it, then move away as you exhale to cool it back down. During sex, avoid muffling or altering your sexual groans and grunts into moans or sighs, which can cause the rhythm of your breath to become unnatural. Instead, take deep full inhales and exhales, and welcome the audible sounds you may make as you do this.

To intensify your orgasms, you can slow down your breath just before you climax and take one deep inhale, imagining energy traveling all the way from your sexual organs up to the top of your head with a giant breath that you "trap" at the top of your head. If you combine this with a contraction of your pelvic musculature, you will often find that it keeps you from experiencing a full orgasm, after which you can exhale and continue the act of lovemaking for a longer period of time. This "tantric sex" tactic is something I learned in *The Multi-Orgasmic Man: Sexual Secrets Every Man Should Know,* which is an excellent companion to David Deida's two books cited above.

Fourth, breathwork (and, incidentally, fasting) pairs perfectly to prayer.

There is a concept in many religions, including Christianity, of spiritual breathing. Like physical breathing, spiritual breathing is a process of "exhaling the impure" and "inhaling the pure." For example, while praying, during an exhale you may confess a sin or release a negative emotion such as shame, anger, or fear; then during the inhale, you can ask God to empower you to release any temptation you may have towards that sin, while "breathing in" or dwelling upon positive emotions such as peace, love, and joy. Or you may simply think or say one small phrase such as "fill me" on the inhale, and then "forgive me" on the exhale. In most cases, spiritual breathing during prayer simply involves some type of confession or release on the exhale, followed by trust, love, and forgiveness on the inhale. You can check out a link I'll include on the resources page for this chapter to learn more about breath prayer as an ancient spiritual practice.

THE BREATH OF LIFE

Finally, and most importantly, breath is integral to life itself.

- I must have read C.S. Lewis' *Chronicles Of Narnia* series nearly a dozen times when I was a boy. In the first book of the series—The Lion, The Witch, and The Wardrobe—Aslan, the King of Narnia, comes across creatures that were transformed into stone statues by a witch. He breathes on them, and they transform from lifeless blocks of stone into sentient, warm-blooded creatures once again. This is a perfect depiction of our own creation as humans: In the book of Genesis, God breathed into the nostrils of the first man Adam, and that was the final step for Adam to become a thinking, feeling creature.

As a matter of fact, the popular phrase "breath of life" comes originally from a verse in Genesis describing this creation of man.

Genesis 2:7 says: *"The Lord God formed the man of dust from the ground and breathed into his nostrils the breath of life, and the man became a living creature."*

In other words, it was a breath from God that transformed us from a lifeless corpse into a living human being. We find this same concept of the breath of life scattered frequently throughout Scripture, including in texts such as:

John 20:22 - *"And with that he breathed on them and said, 'Receive the Holy Spirit.'"* (this Holy Spirit is the same magical elixir that I talk about in Chapter 9.

Job 33:4 - *"The Spirit of God has made me, and the breath of the Almighty gives me life."*

Genesis 2:7 - *"Then the Lord God formed the man of dust from the ground and breathed into his nostrils the breath of life, and the man became a living creature."*

Job 27:3 - *"As long as my breath is in me, and the spirit of God is in my nostrils.."*

Ezekiel 37:6 - *"And I will lay sinews upon you, and will cause flesh to come upon you, and cover you with skin, and put breath in you, and you shall live, and you shall know that I am the Lord."*

Psalms 150:6 - *"Let everything that has breath praise the Lord!'"*

Let everything that has breath praise the Lord, indeed. I am a miracle, you are a miracle, and our bodies - including our respiratory systems - are absolutely also miracles. You should be in awe and thankful for the magical complexity of breath every day. I recommend you begin by silently thanking God with each and every breath that you take when you engage in a daily mindful breathing habit, even if just for one minute. Eventually, this emotion of gratitude will subconsciously become woven into every breath you take.

Summary

Ultimately, I believe that an intimate connection to your own breath is one of the best gifts you can give to yourself, your loved one, or your children.

I'd even go so far as to say that I believe some kind of breath training should ideally be woven into the educational curriculum or parenting protocol for every young human on the planet. I've even taught many of these tactics to my own twin boys, and they can now turn to their breath for sleep, study, meditation, focus, prayer, workouts, and even ice baths.

Finally, if you want to take a deep dive into all things breath, there are a host of helpful podcasts and articles I've published in the past. If you were to pair a digestion of all of these along with the breathwork course I'll include a link to on the resources page for this chapter, you'll be well on your way to becoming a true breath "ninja."

Do you have a breathwork practice? Have you found certain breath resources to be helpful? Do you use your breath to not only enhance your physical and mental health, but also your spiritual health? If not, consider starting today! Despite the extreme importance of your breath, it is here that I cannot resist a bit of a religious pun, specifically by telling you that, despite what many so-called "breatharians" believe, humans "cannot live by breath alone." You'll need actual caloric nourishment too, and in the next chapter, I'll share with you my own perspective on the spiritual side of food.

For resources, references, links and additional reading and listening material for this chapter, visit FitSoulBook.com/Chapter13.

MY FATHER'S WORLD

I recently wrote a cookbook. It's called *The Boundless Cookbook.*

As a result of all my recent writing about food, special ingredients from near and afar, and tinkering in the kitchen, I've been thinking quite a bit about the magic and intricacy woven into the foods and ingredients that we eat. I'd like to share with you several important thoughts I have been having lately about one of my favorite activities: eating.

But allow me to clarify something first: I'm not a chef.

Yes, I'm definitely not a chef. With zero formal training in cooking, I've simply achieved any cooking chops I do have via learning recipes from a mash-up of cooking videos I've come across on YouTube (e.g. random Google searches for terms like "how to make liver taste good"), simple tips my wife mutters as she passes by me in the kitchen while I attempt to make myself a proper meal (e.g. "Babe, add a bit of coconut flour to those salmon cakes and they'll stop crumbling on you!") to insightful tips and tricks from the host of nutrition and cookbooks I read and review on a weekly basis (e.g. mix lemon juice with your bone broth to increase collagen bioavailability).

Sure, I took advanced courses in biochemistry, chemistry, microbiology, physics, and nutrition in college, and I'm sure those have assisted my learning curve in the kitchen quite dramatically, but I will be the first to admit that when it comes to cooking, and especially writing a cookbook, I have full-blown imposter syndrome.

My wife? She's a rancher girl who can, with nary a drip of sweat, whip up a crispy roasted chicken on a Friday night and a batch of mouth-watering sourdough cinnamon rolls on a Saturday morning, all from scratch.

My twin boys? They've been taking cooking classes since they were four years old and can expertly fashion a chocolate souffle and mushroom risotto for their freaking lunch. Heck, they even have their own cooking podcast (GoGreenfields.com) in which they reveal a new taste-bud bursting brainchild each week.

Me? I grew up on boxed macaroni and cheese, 29-cent hamburgers, frozen hot dogs, and whey protein shakes. So for most of my life, I was largely limited to a microwave, a blender, and a drive-thru.

But nonetheless, I do like to tinker in the kitchen. I do like to crack the code on how to use science and spices to unlock nutrients and enhance the digestibility of the vast array of scrumptious foods this planet is blessed with. And as a self-proclaimed foodie, I *definitely* like to eat and I like to eat good food. As a result of my passion for all things food and health, I'm asked with surprising and increasing frequency for all the crazy and unique recipes I frequently mention on podcasts and articles or feature in food porn photos on social media.

So I finally decided to sit down and churn out a cookbook chock full of my favorite recipes—recipes that are mentioned, often with great scientific detail, in my book *Boundless* and across my media platforms (particularly Instagram), but recipes that have never been fully fleshed out in terms of my exact ingredients and preparation strategies. In other words, it's one thing to read in Boundless about how fermenting your own yogurt changes the biome of the gut in a favorable manner and enhances many aspects of endocrine and immune function, but it's quite another matter to know exactly how I wake up in the morning and quickly whip up a batch of homemade yogurt, the methods I use to make the bacteria more concentrated or bioavailable, what I mix it with for goals such as sleep enhancement or muscle building, or even how long the stuff stays good in the refrigerator.

So I obviously think a lot about food, ingredients, spices, herbs, plants, and all manner of things cooking and eating-related, particularly in relation to our own fulfillment and happiness when it comes to our food. As a result, I've had three thoughts jumbling about in my head that I'd like to share with you in this chapter.

First, when you are tinkering in the kitchen with your own recipes, whether new or old, I encourage you to prepare your food mindfully. Take a simple cup of coffee, for example. Sure, you can rush to your kitchen in the morning, grunt or curse as you fumble with the coffee filter, hastily prepare your water as you glance at your watch and think about your email inbox, then hover over your coffee, sipping madly as you scroll through text messages and barely tasting a bean that had to be hauled all the way up from the backwoods of South America to be able to grace your grocery store shelves. Alternatively, you can slowly open the bag of coffee, take a satisfying whiff of an intense aroma of floral and cacao, perk up your ears as listen to the whooshing and light sprinkling of the water as it drizzles into the kettle or coffee maker, and enjoy those first few coffee sips, perhaps with your eyes closed, fully mindful and grateful of a rich superfood from regions beyond that has magically appeared in your kitchen to fire up your precious brain for a day of impactful and purposeful work. *Notice the difference?* Food and drink should be enjoyed with the full array of senses, and prepared and consumed with mindfulness and gratefulness.

Truly, in our tiny pantries and humble kitchens, we now have access to the same cinnamons and spices from the Orient, fruits and beans from the Amazon, and dried berries and cured meats and cheeses from Northern Europe that kings and queens of old would have dished out buckets of gold for and sent out explorers, sailors, and armies on quests to capture and harvest.

As you approach food in this more mindful way, you may, especially if you like music or play a musical instrument, enjoy thinking of it a bit like making music, which is a practice that requires a great deal of mindfulness. Managing multiple pans on the stove is like playing the drums and finely slicing a clove of garlic like tuning a mandolin. *But would you play the drums with a phone cradled to your ear or tune a mandolin while firing off a text message?* Approach food, and even food preparation, similarly.

Second, I encourage you to be in constant awe at the wonders of God's creation. I'm ceaselessly aware of the magic, beauty, mystery, and wonder of the vast array of superfoods scattered across this Earth. Take a variant of the humble buckwheat plant, for example: the Himalayan Tartary Buckwheat, which I just made blueberry pancakes with on last Saturday morning as a surprise for my boys (using a fermentation pancake recipe similar to the one I'll link to on the resources page for this chapter).

Himalayan Tartary Buckwheat (let's call it "HTB" so as not to get too long in the tooth) is a hardy plant that has been farmed in Asia for generations but is largely unknown in the rest of the world. (I had a hard time hunting it down myself, but found a tiny farm in New York State called "Angelica Mills" that grows it.) Modern analyses have revealed that HTB contains significantly higher levels of phytonutrients compared to common buckwheat—up to a 100-fold increase of certain immune-strengthening flavonoids. HTB is also incredibly rich in the flavonoids rutin, quercetin, hesperidin, luteolin, and diosmin. Nutritionally speaking, this portfolio of flavonoids is an orchestra, a symphony, and a masterpiece of the Creator's genius. Each is unique, but together they are wondrous, especially when it comes to the positive ways they can influence immune function.

CHAPTER XIV

Next, 2-hydroxybenzylamine (2-HOBA) is a plant chemical that is extremely rare to find in any foods, but it just so happens that HTB is one of the best sources currently known. 2-HOBA is now being studied for how well it stops the formation of some types of many harmful molecules in the body. Calcium-hydroxy-methyl butyrate monohydrate (yep, that's a mouthful!) is another significant component of HTB. This nutrient, which is found in alfalfa and other foods, has been studied for immune support and rejuvenation, as well as the ways it helps build, maintain, and protect muscles and lean tissues throughout the body. Then there's chlorophyllin, also found in high amounts in HTB. *In plants, chlorophyll turns light into energy.* What can it do for humans? It turns out that it can improve the way the body deals with certain toxins and gets rid of them.

At sufficient levels, chlorophyll can protect DNA and chromosomes, and even help cells repair themselves from damage. Heck, if you read a book like Sayer Ji's *Regenerate* or Arturo Herrera's *The Human Photosynthesis* (both of which are fascinating reads), you can discover how photons of energy from sunlight can actually interact with the chlorophyll in your bloodstream to generate electrons that allow for the production of cellular energy—even in the absence of calories from food!

Just think about it: That's all from one tiny humble buckwheat plant that has been treasured in Asia for thousands of years but that we in the West barely know anything about (though we've certainly cracked the code on how to genetically modify wheat and spray it with herbicides and pesticides to make a relatively nutrient-void frankenplant for our hamburger buns!). Multitudes of other examples abound, examples that display the mysteries and wonders of superfoods in Creation. From Goji berries and coffeeberry fruit, to spirulina and chlorella algae, to Barùkas nuts and chia seeds, we walk a planet rich in bountiful blessings. Yet how often do we drop our jaws in pure awe at these mysterious, wonderful fruits of the Earth?

In the Bible, Psalms 104:24-25 sums up the wonders of our Father's world quite nicely:

> *"O Lord, how manifold are your works!*
> *In wisdom have you made them all;*
> *the earth is full of your creatures.*
> *Here is the sea, great and wide,*
> *which teems with creatures innumerable,*
> *living things both small and great."*

Elsewhere, in John 3:1, we learn that *"All things were made by him; and without him* was not anything made that was made." So yes, that means that an Almighty God formed and fashioned the cacao tree, the cannabis plant, the chickpea, and the catfish—and all this marvelous bounty is ours to enjoy in all of its intricacy, beauty and, yes, tastiness.

Wait...*everything?*

Even *meat*—which technically involves blood, killing, and a loss of life?

This is an interesting idea to unpack, so let's take a brief foray. After all, I'm often asked how I, as a Christian, could condone the shedding of the blood of an animal and the subsequent eating of that animal's meat, especially if human-kind was originally created in a beautiful, lush garden chock full of enough highly nutritious and edible plants and vegetables that could theoretically sustain life in the absence of carnivory.

It's certainly true that in the Creation story of Genesis in the Bible, God created man (Adam) and woman (Eve) and put them in a garden (Eden). Furthermore, it does indeed appear that the original form of sustenance meant for humankind was comprised of plant-based foods, such as fruits and vegetables, seeds, nuts, and trees.

For example...

...Genesis 1:29-30 says: *"Then God said, "I give you every seed-bearing plant on the face of the whole earth and every tree that has fruit with seed in it. They will be yours for food. And to all the beasts of the earth and all the birds in the sky and all the creatures that move along the ground—everything that has the breath of life in it—I give every green plant for food." And it was so."*

...Genesis 2:7-9: *"And the Lord God formed man of the dust of the ground, and breathed into his nostrils the breath of life, and man became a living soul. And the Lord God planted a garden eastward of Eden, and there he put the man whom he had formed. And out of the ground made the Lord God to grow every tree that is pleasant to the sight, and good for food..."*

...and Genesis 2:15-16: *"And the Lord God took the man and put him into the Garden of Eden to dress it and to keep it. And the Lord God commanded the man, saying, of every tree of the garden thou mayest freely eat..."*

So arguably, since death and killing would not have existed prior to Adam and Eve committing sin and bringing death upon this planet, then the necessary shedding of blood via meat-eating did not exist, and furthermore, God instructed His original human creation to consume a pure, 100% plant-based, vegan diet.

However, elsewhere in the Bible, it appears that the eating of meat or consumption of animal-based products becomes both necessary and acceptable.

For example, anyone familiar with Christianity has undoubtedly heard the Promised Land being referred to as "a land flowing with milk and honey." That phrase "a land flowing with milk and honey" actually appears 20 times in the Bible—Exodus 3:8, Exodus 3:17, Exodus 13:5, Exodus 33:3, Leviticus 20:24, Numbers 13:27, Numbers 14:8, Numbers 16:13, Numbers 16:14, Deuteronomy 6:3, Deuteronomy 11:9, Deuteronomy 26:9, Deuteronomy 26:15, Deuteronomy 27:3, Deuteronomy 31:20, Joshua 5:6, Jeremiah 11:5, Jeremiah 32:22, Ezekiel 20:6, and Ezekiel 20:15! Of course, both milk and honey are animal-based foods dependent on some form of animal and insect domestication for the harvesting of those foods.

Furthermore, meat is often referenced as an acceptable food source in the Bible, including in passages such as:

1 Corinthians 10:25: *"Eat whatever is sold in the meat market without raising any question on the ground of conscience."*

Acts 10:9-16: *"The next day, as they were on their journey and approaching the city, Peter went up on the housetop about the sixth hour to pray. And he became hungry and wanted something to eat, but while they were preparing it, he fell into a trance and saw the heavens opened and something like a great sheet descending, being let down by its four corners upon the earth. In it were all kinds of animals and reptiles and birds of the air. And there came a voice to him: "Rise, Peter; kill and eat." ...*

Luke 24:41-43: *"And while they yet believed not for joy, and wondered, he [Jesus] said unto them, Have ye here any meat? And they gave him a piece of a broiled fish, and of a honeycomb. And he took it, and did eat before them."*

Perhaps two of the best examples of God's approval of eating meat comes A) from the celebration of the Passover, in which each Israelite family was commanded to take a lamb or goat, kill it, and put its blood on the doorposts, then to eat the meat by morning, and burn the leftovers before daybreak, and B) the fact that many of the early disciples were fishermen, the frequent consumption of fish within the New Testament, and most notably, Luke 24:41-43, which explicitly says that Jesus asked for food and that he thankfully ate fish and honey which the disciples gave him.

Now, that all being said, my own perspective on this frequently debated topic is that at one time, the Earth was pristine, free of sin, pollution, and toxicity; and there was also a pre-great Flood atmosphere that ensured highly nutritious plant matter derived from fruits, vegetables, seeds, and nuts of a completely different and more nutrient-dense nature than modern-day plants and agriculture. As a result, the original human creation was likely equipped to do just fine on a plant-based diet. The pre-flood atmosphere of the earth was likely far different than our living conditions today, possibly providing more oxygen and greater protection against the excess UVA and UVB radiation from the sun, and greater abundance and nutrient density of plants and fruit-bearing trees.

However, things seem to have changed. After the flood, it is possible that fruits and vegetables became smaller and/or more scarce (Genesis 8:22 says that *"...as long as the earth endures, seedtime and harvest, cold and heat, summer and winter, day and night will never cease."*). Omnivory became permissible and acceptable, and probably even necessary for adequate nutrient, vitamin, and calorie availability. God fed the Israelites in the desert with not just manna from heaven, but also with thousands of quail. Agriculture also sprung forth, and bread, along with wheat, barley, beans, lentils, millet, and spelt are often mentioned in Scripture (much to the chagrin of many Paleo diet enthusiasts, who seem to think gluten is a demonic protein from hell!).

One day, when heaven and earth are restored to their pristine conditions, this scenario may all change. There will likely no longer be a need for death, bloodshed, or meat consumption. Isaiah 11:6-9 gives us clues about this when it says:

> *"The wolf shall dwell with the lamb, and the leopard shall lie down with the young goat, and the calf and the lion and the fattened calf together; and a little child shall lead them. The cow and the bear shall graze; their young shall lie down together; and the lion shall eat straw like the ox. The nursing child shall play over the hole of the cobra, and the weaned child shall put his hand on the adder's den. They shall not hurt or destroy in all my holy mountain; for the earth shall be full of the knowledge of the Lord as the waters cover the sea."*

So ultimately, to come full circle: yes, I believe all of God's creation is here for our culinary enjoyment and sustenance, and that includes all plants and animals from cabbages to cows, carrots to clams, parsnips to pork, and flax to fish.

Finally, and *third* (after that hefty rabbit hole above!) I encourage you to enjoy your food in a parasympathetic state of relaxation, mindfulness, and gratefulness. Quickly sucking down your smoothie hunched over a steering wheel as you stressfully navigate on your morning commute or wiping smoothie shards off your face while fumbling with the music dial on the car is a far, far different experience—both psychologically and physiologically—compared to sitting at your kitchen table in the sunshine, savoring every bite, and perhaps jotting down a few notes in your gratitude journal, thumbing through your favorite magazine, or chatting with your family. Eating in a stressed state predisposes you to leaky gut syndrome, inadequate digestive enzyme production, poor nutrient absorption, and overeating—all topics I explore in great detail in the "How To Fix Your Gut" chapter of my book *Boundless*. In contrast, eating in a relaxed state, often with friends and family, usually in between and not during bouts of work or commuting, allows you to savor and enjoy your food, digest your food, and feel more satiated from each and every bite that you mindfully chew.

In fact, research has shown that to truly digest your meal, get the maximum nutritional benefit from the food and experience the minimum inflammatory impact on the gut, an average number of 25-40 times per bite is what you should aim for when chewing your food (you learn plenty more tips about oral care, jaw strength and how to breathe/chew properly in the "Beauty & Symmetry" chapter of *Boundless*). This savoring and gratefulness for food can ultimately bring us closer to our Creator.

So as trite as a bite of a wild apple may seem, or a routine as a ho-hum meat and potatoes dinner may seem or as functional as an energy drink or bar we might suck down or munch on during a workout may seem, any dietary practice can bring us closer to our greatest purpose in life if we approach it with the right mentality—by consuming it in full gratitude to fuel our hearts with the joy and love of God, as Paul so eloquently states in his letter to the Corinthians in the Bible:

"So whether you eat or drink or whatever you do, do it all to the glory of God."

John Piper also sums this up quite nicely in his excellent book *Don't Waste Your Life* when he says:

> *"God created you and me to live with a single all-embracing all-transforming passion - namely a passion to glorify God by enjoying and displaying his supreme excellence in all the spheres of life."*

And yes, that supreme excellence in all spheres of life includes swinging a kettlebell and making a superfood smoothie.

In my own personal experience, I've found that one of the best ways to approach each meal with this spirit of mindfulness, gratitude, and relaxation is to create some kind of routine or ritual for each meal. This pre-meal habit can include a few relaxing breaths, a blessing, a prayer, or even a song.

For example, one easy breathwork practice we often do at the dinner table is to simply close the eyes, take a deep, slow breath in through the nose, then out through slightly pursed lips and repeat three times. Another simple habit is to think of one thing you're grateful for and say it aloud prior to your meal; or if you are in a group, you can go around the table and have each person name one thing they are grateful for. Or you can say a simple prayer and bless the food. In addition to thanking God for providing yet another blessing of nutrients, calories, and sustenance, I also like this pleasant twist on a Thich Nhat Hanh blessing, which I learned from a friend at an immersive health event I teach at called RUNGA. It goes like this:

> *"Breathing in, I'm aware of my body.*
> *Breathing out, I smile at my body.*
> *Breathing In, I am aware of my food.*
> *Breathing out, I smile at my food.*
> *Breathing in, I'm aware of my company.*
> *Breathing out, I smile at my company."*

An entire group gathered around a table can do this together, eyes closed, breathing in and out together as one person leads and the others repeat the words that person recites.

Does all this seem to make it sound to you like there's a deep spiritual aspect to food?

You would be correct if you suspected so. After all, food isn't just about minerals, vitamins, proteins, carbohydrates, fat, and calories. Food connects us. Food fuels traditions and memories. Food is something we gather around. Food changes our mood, for better or worse. Food can create bliss and contentment that one feels far beyond their stomach, small intestine, large intestine, and bloodstream. *Food can feed the fit soul.* Do not underestimate the invisible energy and frequency contained within each bite that you eat, and the impact of your own energy and frequency on each bite you eat.

So when our own Greenfield family finishes a hard day jam-packed with work, chores, school, phone calls, consults, meetings, emails, workouts, animal care, podcasts, articles, books and we all finally gather around the dining room table to breathe in the sweet aroma of a salted, roasted chicken with baked carrot fries and fresh sprouts drenched in extra virgin olive oil and dressed with crumbled goat cheese, and I take that first sip of dark, rich organic wine, a smile erupts on my face, and also in my soul— not only because of the deep, intense sense of relaxation and pleasure I derive from gathering around a beautiful cornucopia of aromatic food with my precious family, but also because I know I helped grow those sprouts from tiny alfalfa, red clover, and broccoli seeds and had a chance to participate in the magic of growing, nourishing, and savoring God's creation.

As you begin yourself to ponder the wonders of God's Creation, think about the well-known Christian hymn "This Is My Father's World", which is one of my favorite poetic declarations of the wonders of this universe in which we exist, and also a marvelous song to sing or listen to prior to any meal:

> "This is my Father's World
> And to my listening ears
> All nature sings and round me rings
> The music of the spheres
> This is my Father's world
> I rest me in the thought
> Of rocks and trees
> Of skies and seas
> His hands the wonders rod
> This is my Father's world
> The birds there carols raise
> The morning light the lily white
> Declare their maker's praise
> This is my Father's world
> He shines in all that's fair
> In rustling grass I hear him pass
>
> He speaks to me everywhere
> This is my Father's world
> And to my listening ears
> All nature sings and round me rings
> The music of the sphere."

Based on that, here's one final idea for you: the next time you are preparing to eat or gathering your family and friends around a table for breakfast, lunch or dinner, simply play or sing this song and dwell upon the words. Then say a prayer of gratefulness, smile and "dig into" God's creation with full mindfulness and joy. Incidentally, the positive emotions that will pour forth into your life are the very same emotions that, if absent, can result in the type of health "issues" you're about to discover in the next chapter.

For resources, references, links and additional reading and listening material for this chapter, visit FitSoulBook.com/Chapter14.

CHAPTER XV

BONES OF STEEL

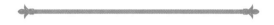

My wife is a skinny, Montana rancher girl who is tough and hard, but also has what I would consider to be thin "bird bones" along with a slight, lean build that—if not kept strong via loading along the long axis of the bone, high mineral intake, omega-3 fatty acids, fat-soluble vitamins, DHEA and progesterone optimization and plenty of the other tactics I tackle in a very thorough osteoporosis podcast episode I'll link to on the resources page for this chapter—could very well increase her risk for developing a high amount of frailty and fragility as she ages, resulting in the possibility of her doing something like fracturing a hip if she steps off a curb the wrong way when she's 60 years old.

I, of course, care for and love my wife, so I'm careful to (in a "non-nagging" sort of way) ensure that she tends to her bones so that any genetic risk for osteoporosis or osteopenia is nipped in the bud and does not manifest.

But no matter how many kettlebell squats she does, how much calcium and vitamin K she consumes, and how much caffeine and alcohol she avoids in her quest for bones of steel, she's also—based on the studying up we've done on folks like Bruce Lipton (author of *Biology Of Belief*) and David Hawkins (author of *Healing & Recovery*) and above all, the Bible—careful to focus on releasing any feelings of anger, hate, selfishness or bitterness in her life, all of which are associated with, you guessed it, bone "issues."

For example, in Chinese traditional medicine, the emotion of anger is not only associated with bone cancer, but the disturbance of several other emotions (especially melancholy, anxiety, and anger) is also considered to significantly contribute to the pathogenesis of chronic disease. You're going to learn plenty more about that shortly.

It All Began In Northern Galilee

But let's begin here...

...I first realized the power of emotions and stress to affect disease risk when I traveled to Israel for a tour of the country's unique collection of health spas, fitness centers, healing retreats, and wellness facilities. While there, in Northern Galilee, I visited the home of a former professional basketball player – Doron Sheffer (who I interviewed in a heart moving podcast called Why You Get Cancer & What To Do About It, *which I'll link to on the resources page for this chapter).*

Doron had been an amazing athlete.

He was an achiever.

A hard-charger.

A "professional person."

As a guard for the dominant college basketball team UConn, he fed the ball to star teammates like Ray Allen and played for legendary coach Jim Calhoun. Sheffer averaged five assists and thirteen points per game, he hit 40% of his three-point attempts, and led the Uconn Huskies to a brilliant 89-13 record, along with NCAA tournament appearances in each of his three seasons. He then became the first Israeli ever drafted by the NBA when the Los Angeles Clippers selected him in the second round in 1996, but he instead signed a lucrative contract with the Israeli professional basketball team, Maccabi Tel Aviv, which he then led to four consecutive national championships.

But then Doron got testicular cancer. When I sat down with him in his backyard garden looking over the beautiful hills of Amirim, eating a meal of organic figs, goji berries, and sweet local almonds, he described to me how the tremendous pressure, tension, difficulties, frustrations, pent-up emotions, and stress from the life of a hard-charging professional athlete eventually built up inside him and culminated in disease.

Indeed, scientists have actually discovered that emotional stress similar to what Doron experienced can be a trigger for the growth of tumors. **As a matter of fact, any sort of trauma, emotional or physical stress, can act as a literal pathway between cancerous mutations, bringing them together in a potentially fatal combination. For example, at Yale University,** scientists have now discovered **that everyday emotional**

stress is a trigger for the growth of tumors. The findings show that the conditions for developing cancer can be significantly affected by your emotional environment, including everyday work and family stress. In other words, your risk of developing cancer can be positively or negatively affected by your emotional environment, including everyday work, physical, emotional, and relationship stress.

The traditional Chinese medical view of cancer etiology has long-held that emotions are a major contributing factor for cancer. For example, author Sun Binyan writes in his book Cancer Treatment and Prevention:

> *"According to our understanding of the tumor patient, most have suppression of the emotions. They tend to hold in their anger. Although some patients have good results after treatment, emotional stimulation may cause them to decline again, and then the previous treatment would have been in vain. Some people have a severe phobia about cancer. Before they know the real disease, they have a lot of suspicion. Once they know they have cancer, their whole spirit breaks down. This kind of spiritual state is very bad for the treatment."*

In the book, *Prevention and Treatment of Carcinoma in Traditional Chinese Medicine,* Jia Kun gives ten recommendations for cancer prevention. In addition to a good environment and personal hygiene, proper amounts of physical activity and rest, good eating habits and healthy food, and avoiding smoking, he states that:

"Emotional changes, such as worry, fear, hesitation, anger, irritation, and nervousness should be prevented. Mental exhaustion is harmful and life should be enriched with entertainment."

Chinese medicine authors Shi Lanling and Shi Peiquan also mention the etiology of various cancers in their book *Experience in Treating Carcinomas with Traditional Chinese Medicine:*

> *"The etiologic factors of the disease involve chiefly the disturbance of the seven emotions, especially melancholy, anxiety, and anger, which are liable to impair the spleen and the liver. Impaired by melancholy and anxiety, qi will be stagnated and the spleen will lose the function of transformation and transportation, leading to disturbance of water metabolism and the subsequent accumulation of phlegm-dampness, while, impaired by anger, the liver qi will be*

stagnated. The stagnated liver qi, as qi is the commander of blood,
may give rise to blood stasis if not relieved in time. Thus, emotional
disturbance, in-coordination between the ascending-descending
movement of qi of the zang-fu organs, sluggish flow of qi and blood,
and the ensuing obstruction of dampness, phlegm, and blood stasis
are the fundamental pathogenesis of the disease."

In their section on treatment of breast cancer, the authors refer to a discussion in a Ming Dynasty text by the surgeon Chen Shigong (1555-1636 A.D.) that indicates that breast cancer "results from anxiety, emotional depression, and overthinking which impairs the liver, spleen, and heart and causes the obstruction of the channels." This text is also mentioned in *The Treatment of Cancer by Integrated Chinese-Western Medicine,* and is translated as follows:

"Breast cancer is due to worry and melancholy. Lots of ideas
hanging around make one feel dissatisfied. Perverse flow of liver qi
to the spleen leads to the obstruction of the channels and collaterals
and congelations due to excessive accumulation."

In addition, the book *Cancer Treatment with Fu Zheng Pei Ben Principle* presents a section on the etiology of cancer, and describes the following with regards to emotional disturbances:

"TCM (Traditional Chinese Medicine) embodies changes of spirit
and sentiment as the seven emotions: pleasure, anger, grief, fear,
yearning, sorrow, surprise, all of which are emotional,
physiological reactions of an organism towards external changes in
its environment. Emotional disturbance refers to reactions, either
excessive (excitation) or insufficient (inhibition) which will
ultimately lead to disturbances in the flowing of qi and blood and
the visceral functions, with subsequent illness. TCM claims rage
harms the liver, excessive stimulation harms the heart, grief harms
the spleen, great sorrow harms the lungs, and fear harms the
kidneys. Though not necessarily precise, this belief definitely points
out that emotional injury will affect the physiological functions of
the qi, blood, viscera, and channels, and lower the body resistance,
resulting in disease. The human body is susceptible to cancer when
under emotional stress or disturbance."

One major study published in China involving a significant population of approximately 750,000 individuals in Beijing attempted to determine if psychosocial factors contributed to the incidence of primary lung cancer. They reported three factors positively associated with lung cancer: 1) a burst of emotion that could not be controlled; 2) poor working circumstances, including poor relationships with co-workers; and 3) a depressive feeling for a long time.

Western research, in a field termed "Affective Immunology," has gone on to support the idea that depression can impair immune system functions. For example, it has been shown that tumor-relevant lymphocyte subpopulations, also known as natural killer cells (NK cells, which can attack cancer cells), have receptors for various neuropeptide proteins, including those released during stress. This means that NK cell activity can be influenced by emotions. The level of NK cell activity has been shown in research to be a good predictor of breast cancer outcome, and a loss of NK activity in cancer patients has been shown to be correlated with psychosocial measures such as the level of patient adjustment (avoiding showing distress at the cancer diagnosis or treatment - such as internalizing the stress), lack of social support, and symptoms of fatigue or depression (incidentally, laughing and joy has been shown to increase NK activity).

If you read a book such as *The Healing Code* or look into the vast amount of research on the link between emotional stress and chronic disease, much of which I'll include on the resources page for this chapter, you'll see hundreds of examples of how the sympathetic nervous system (SNS), the fight-or-flight portion of the nervous system, can actually encourage metastasis when chronically elevated. During acute stress, the SNS becomes active. But as soon as a stressful event has passed, the body returns back to homeostasis within about an hour. But under chronic stress, the SNS is turned on virtually all the time, and in this chronically stressed state, adrenaline and noradrenaline can alter genetic expression via the same protein-folding mechanisms you've already discovered in this chapter. This genetic alteration can lead to a number of pro-cancer processes, including activation of inflammatory responses, inhibition of immune responses and programmed cancer cell death, reduction in the cytotoxic function of NK cells, inhibition of DNA repair, stimulation of cancer cell angiogenesis, and activation of epithelial-mesenchymal transition, which is one of the ways new cancer stem cells are created.

One researcher, Dr. Harold Burr, used mice to determine if the energy field of the human body can play a role in cancer. He measured the energy fields of the mice fields and noted which mice later developed cancer. After taking more than 10,000 measurements, he found that the electromagnetic signature of cancer appeared in the mouse's energy field before any detectable cellular malignancy was even evident! Burr also looked at a group of healthy women who did not have a diagnosis of uterine cancer. Interestingly, the women who had an electromagnetic signature for uterine cancer - even though they were apparently healthy - were the ones who went on to develop cancer later. In other words, cancer was showing up in the field of energy before it showed up in the physical cells!

Burr's body of work demonstrates the wisdom of an ancient saying in traditional Chinese medicine: "The mind controls the qi, and the blood follows the qi." The ancient sages were referring to life energy, and by blood they meant the matter of the body. Energy influences matter! Perhaps this is why research has shown tumors shrinking to less than half their original size within just a few hours of an emotional therapy session that elicited positive healing emotions, why studies have shown the DNA in cancer cells in Petri dishes in labs disintegrate when positive emotions were directed to those cells by Chinese traditional medical practitioners, and why mindfulness meditation for just three months has been shown to induce an anti-aging effect by directly growing your telomeres.

Now here's the deal: I'm personally a hard-charging guy focused on personal and professional excellence in everything I do. But I truly believe that unless you are able to relax, breathe, de-stress, and simply stop and smell the roses, you're going to be the kind of person who eventually develops a chronic-stress related disease that forces your fast-forward life into slow-motion. So you have to put the brakes on before your body puts the brakes on and forces you to stop, perhaps with the flu, perhaps with back pain, or perhaps with cancer. Make sense?

The ultimate question is: How can you do this?

How can you slow down before your body forces you to slow down?

How can you somehow dig yourself out of a hole of a constant barrage of emails, text messages, phone calls, over-exercising, eating to train and training to eat, going to bed late, 24-7 self-quantified biohacking, trying to have everything, FOMO, getting up early, and still somehow managing to squeeze in some semblance of quality in your friend and family relationships?

This is exactly what Doron figured out, and this man's new approach to life, his answers, and his new aura of peace and calm spoke heavily to me when I interviewed him. He defied conventional medicine and naturally healed his body of cancer, and his approach to life is now refreshing, relaxed, and incredibly peaceful. When I visited

Doron at his peaceful home and private health resort Hyuli in Amirim, in the mountains of Northern Israel, I was surrounded by a laid-back, de-stressed community of aromatherapists, massage therapists, herb gardens, spas, a health food shop, an organic olive oil shop, art galleries, restaurants, and wellness bed and breakfasts. These mountains are where Doron slipped away from chronic stress, reinvigorated his body, and underwent his own spiritual cleanse to win his battle against testicular cancer.

In short, Doron healed himself by radically changing his environment and emotions.

The Biology Of Your Beliefs

Now I could stop here, but I know that many of my readers dig the "hardcore science" so to speak, or at least may like to delve into some of the chemical, genetic, and physical factors underlying this link between emotions and physical health. So put on your thinking caps, because we're about to delve into a few of the concepts that stem cell biologist and author Bruce Lipton, Ph.D. shares in his highly relevant book *The Biology of Belief: Unleashing the Power of Consciousness, Matter & Miracles.*

In the book, and often during his speeches, Bruce shares a quote from Albert Einstein:

> *"The field is the sole governing agency of the particle."*

Dr. Lipton claims that if we can prove that our thoughts can create that "field" and if the field is what actually controls and governs the particle (physical matter, our bodies, and the world around us), then what Einstein was actually saying was that our thoughts and intentions can directly create the world that we live in.

So in 1982 (when I was one year old!), Dr. Lipton began examining the principles of quantum physics and how they might be integrated into an understanding of the cell's information processing systems. He proceeded to produce breakthrough studies on the cell membrane, which revealed that this outer layer of the cell was an organic homolog of a computer chip: the cell's equivalent of a brain. His research at Stanford University's School of Medicine went on to reveal that the environment, operating through the electrochemical gradient across the cellular membrane, can control the behavior and physiology of the cell, and even turn genes on and off.

In a nutshell, Lipton teaches that if you have a belief, then the function of the mind is to manifest that belief so it becomes a reality.

For example, if you have a belief that you're going to get a cold because you were around a friend with the sniffles, then the function of the mind is to convert that belief—along with all the anxiety and worry about getting sick and missing a workday or trip to the beach—into physical manifestation, and voila, the next day you wake up with a cold. If you have a strong emotion, positive or negative, around a certain belief, it can cause that particular belief to become your physical reality. According to Lipton, the science of epigenetics is not the science of being defined by your genes or environment but is instead the science of understanding how your interpretation of your life events and environment affects the cells of your physical body.

Seems like a stretch? Maybe not so much a stretch as you would think. See, there is a new scientific awareness of Dr. Lipton's work - an awareness very much related to the genome project, genetic engineering, and the infatuation with DNA that seems to be currently capturing all the media's and health world's attention. To understand this awareness, we must begin with an understanding of how our entire biological lives are driven and managed by proteins, the molecular building blocks of our bodies.

There are over 150,000 different proteins that make up your body. Each protein is a long, linear molecule of amino acids linked end-to-end, and each molecule is like a tiny spine in which the amino acid molecules are miniature vertebrae. There are twenty different amino acids, and each has a unique shape. The final shape of each protein's spine is determined by the specific sequence of each of these uniquely-shaped amino acid links. Ultimately, this means that every cell in your body is built from an assembly of thousands of different-shaped protein molecules.

The novelty of these proteins is that they can change their shape. As a matter of fact, the movement of the protein's tiny spine is analogous to the movement of a human spine. In your own spine, each of the jointed segments can rotate and flex at the point at which they are coupled. On the human spine, it is skeletal muscles that cause this movement. But on the protein spine, movement and shape configuration changes are the result of a repulsive or attractive force generated by electromagnetic fields.

As a protein's electric charge or field is altered, that protein adjusts the shape of its spine to accommodate these forces. When it changes shape from one configuration to another, the protein molecule moves, along with the movement of all the other protein molecules surrounding it, cooperating in functional assemblies called pathways. Respiratory pathways, digestive pathways, and muscle contraction pathways are all examples of assemblies of proteins whose coordinated movements produce specific biological functions.

Studies have now shown that this change in the shape of proteins can actually change the expression of our genetics, and vice versa. Since proteins are altered by electromagnetic fields, including fields generated by thoughts, feelings, and emotions, then this means that genes can be turned on and off by those same fields. That's right: you can control gene activity by focusing on your beliefs. These beliefs, true or false, positive or negative, creative or destructive, exist not only in your mind, but instead influence the very cells of your body. This also means that DNA does not by itself control your biology, and that information can be transmitted throughout your body, to other people's bodies, and even to your descendants in ways other than through the base sequence of DNA.

This means that thoughts, emotions, and energy can activate or inhibit a cell's function-producing proteins, that harnessing the power of your mind can be just as effective or more effective than pharmaceuticals, supplements, and biohacks, and that your perception of your environment is significantly responsible for your health and biological function. What we think, feel, and say, who we are around, and everything in our environment has a significant influence on who we are and how we function, even down to the details of how our genes are expressed.

So is it true that a sunny outlook means fewer colds and less heart disease, hope can somehow protect against hypertension, diabetes, and respiratory tract infections, and happier people live longer? It turns out that research on the biology of emotion - and what it may teach us about helping people to live longer - has been studied at institutions such as Harvard. Laura Kubzansky of the Harvard School of Public Health is at the forefront of such research. In a 2007 study that followed more than 6,000 men and women aged 25 to 74 for 20 years, she found that emotional vitality (a sense of enthusiasm, hopefulness, engagement in life, and ability to face life's stresses with emotional balance) significantly reduces the risk of coronary heart disease, even when accounting for healthy behaviors such as not smoking and regular exercise.

A vast amount of additional scientific literature details how negative emotions harm the body, and how sustained stress or fear can alter biology in a way that, over time, adds up to wear and tear and, eventually, illnesses including heart disease, stroke, and diabetes. For example, chronic anger and anxiety have been proven to disrupt cardiac function by changing the heart's electrical stability, hastening atherosclerosis, and increasing systemic inflammation.

Even the sustained activation of the body's stress response system resulting from early life experiences such as neglect, violence, or living alone with a parent suffering severe mental illness has harmful effects on the brain and other organ systems. But additional research has shown that certain personality traits help people avoid or healthfully manage diseases such as heart attacks, strokes, diabetes, and depression, including emotional vitality (a sense of enthusiasm, hopefulness, and engagement), optimism (a perspective that good things will happen, and that one's actions account for the good things that occur in life), supportive networks of family and friends, and bouncing back from stressful challenges and knowing that things will eventually look up again.

Among dozens of published papers outlining these types of stress responses, Kubzansky has shown that children who are able to stay focused on a task and have a more positive outlook at age 7 report better general health and fewer illnesses as much as 30 years later. She has also found that optimism cuts the risk of heart disease in half!

WHERE QUANTUM BIOLOGY FITS IN

It turns out that some of these phenomena can be explained by the field of quantum biology. I first became familiarized with the ins and outs of quantum biology when I read the fascinating book *The Quantum Doctor"* by Dr. Amit Goswami, who also stars in the equally excellent film on quantum healing entitled *"What The Bleep Do We Know?*

In the book, Dr. Goswami explains how the vibration of the atoms that make up our bodies can have profound effects on our mental and physical well-being. Newtonian mechanics merely recognize the role of chemical signals, such as hormones, growth factors, neurotransmitters, peptides or drugs, and deny the role of the immaterial or unseen energy fields. But energy and vibrational waves, operating through widely accepted quantum mechanics principles and influenced by beliefs and emotions, are just as effective in signaling protein movement as physical chemicals.

The quickest way to begin wrapping your head around this is with a thought experiment.

Pause to take a look at yourself in a mirror, or perhaps the selfie camera on your smartphone. Or just stare at your hand. What do you see?

You see a human being, a single physical individual. But take this further. Under this skin, there's a collection of tissue, muscle, bones, organs, and blood. The truth is, when you see a single individual looking back at you, it's a misperception. Go deeper. What makes up those bones, those muscles, the blood? Cells. And what are cells composed of? Molecules? And then what? Atom particles. When you go inside the atom, at this level you find protons, neutrons, electrons. And taken to the final extent, what are these particles made of?

At this fundamental quantum level, the answer discovered is that there's nothing physical at all. It's all energy and vibration. Looked at from this final perspective, what you see looking back at you in the mirror is the physical expression of energy, and those energy vibrations are influenced by thought patterns, emotions, beliefs, and everything else you're reading about in this article.

Quantum theory states that when the mind observes a set of circumstances or phenomena, it has an impact on the outcome. This is called the observer effect, which, in basic terms, means that if you try to observe a particle, it will act as a particle, and in the absence of observation, it tends to act more like a wave. In the same way, the impact the mind will have upon any physical or mental outcome will be determined by the state of mind of the observer.

In the field of quantum biology, the mind is the primary instrument used to heal the body. The mind of the healer (yourself or another) must be in a healthy state if it is to have a healing effect on the body.

So when the mind is in a state of stress, it will have a negative impact upon the body, which can create illness or disease, but when the mind is in a state of appreciation and well-being, it will have a positive effect upon the body and can result in healing.

In a nutshell, the fields of quantum biology and quantum healing are based around this concept of quantum physics—that your state of mind can actually affect the vibration of molecules in our body, and this can then affect our physical and mental well-being.

THE MAP OF CONSCIOUSNESS

• Two years after meeting with Doron, I discovered the work of Dr. David Hawkins, author of the book *Healing & Recovery*. In his book, Dr. Hawkins describes how to identify protein-shifting and cellular membrane influencing emotions that are either helpful or deleterious, including practical ways to permanently change negative emotions such as anger, shame, and fear, along with how to shift into positive emotions such as peace, love, and joy.

Like Dr. Bruce Lipton, Dr. Hawkins teaches that the body expresses and is subject to what is held in mind, and therefore, the greater the amount of negativity held in the mind, the greater the deleterious effect of this negative energy field on the biological well-being. In contrast, the greater the positive energy, the more positive the health outcomes. It turns out that each emotion, positive or negative, is associated with a specific vibratory frequency that can be measured. For example, at a frequency of about 540Hz, the body can begin to heal from the inside out due to a release of endorphins within the brain.

Let's take a closer look at how emotion can create a specific vibratory frequency. If you've ever opened a physics book, you've probably seen a wave. One cycle of a wave is referred to as a frequency, and frequencies are measured in Hertz (Hz), or the number of waves per second, which means one wave cycle in one second would be one Hz. A high frequency would involve lots of waves per second, while a low frequency would involve just a few cycles per second.

The height of a wave can also be measured and is referred to as voltage (not to be confused with amplitude, which is simply the measurement of the maximum value of the voltage). A wave can be high voltage or low voltage. In addition, the power of a wave is called amperage: waves can have plenty of power behind them (high amp waves with high amplitude), or little power behind them (low amp waves with low amplitude). In addition, a wave's vibration can be smooth or angular, and a wave can have a regular pattern or an irregular pattern. Ultimately the combination of the speed, height, power, smoothness, and regularity of a wave are used to define the vibration of the wave. In other words, vibration is the resulting pattern of all the variables of a wave. As you can imagine, there are billions of combinations of these functions.

Now, here's what's important to understand: Every object on the face of the planet, from the simplest molecule to a tiny mouse to an enormous elephant to your own body has its own unique vibrational fingerprint, a fingerprint created from the infinite combinations of vibrations.

Some physical objects have lower and slower vibrations and some higher and faster vibrations. For example, the book *Molecules of Emotion* by Dr. Candace Pert highlights how molds, viruses, bacteria, and parasites vibrate at around 77 kHz (kilohertz), goldfish at 1,000 kHz, and a human body at 1,520 kHz.

In her book, Dr. Pert highlights how emotions have unique vibrations just like colors and physical objects do. These emotional vibrations also range from higher and faster to lower and slower. For example, when you are laughing and full of joy, your vibrations become higher and faster. When you are tired or sick, your vibrations slow and lower. Recall the last time you fell in love. Did you feel energized and high, as though you were walking on a cloud? That's because your entire body was literally vibrating at a higher frequency. This is also why when you're negative, depressed or stressed, you can feel sluggish, slow, and heavy - your vibrations are lower and slower. This is all scientifically measurable, with much of the latest research performed and measured on power spectrum graphs by the HeartMath Institute, as well as by Kirlian photography. It is possible to take these pictures and measure the human body's frequencies because, as you've already learned, human beings are composed of electromagnetic energy.

Using similar techniques, Dr. David Hawkins has actually measured the vibrational frequency of specific emotions, and, over 20 years of research, kinesiology, and muscle testing, translated these frequencies into a logarithmic scale, along with 17 different levels of consciousness associated with each emotion in what he calls a "Map Of Consciousness."

In his book, he describes how stress proneness and vulnerability are directly related to our current state of emotional vibration. The highest attainable level of consciousness is enlightenment (at 1000). Moving from the 0 to the 1000 mark represents a shift in emotions from the lowest emotion of fear all the way up to the highest emotion of love. Here is how Hawkins describes the different levels of consciousness.

1. *Shame - 1-20: Associated with humiliation, low self-esteem, and paranoia. Someone at this level often feels worthless, and sometimes becomes a rigid or neurotic perfectionist or moral extremist. The life view of this state is misery.*

2. *Guilt - 30: Guilt is accompanied by feelings of blame and remorse, often accompanied by manipulative tendencies and a tendency to be condemning of self and others.*

3. *Apathy - 50: This is a state of helplessness and despair, along with neediness and dependency on others. Because this level of energy feels heavy and burdensome, many people avoid those vibrating at these levels, and some societies even tuck away or hide the poor and homeless who often live at this level. This level is also associated with hopelessness and abdication (giving up one's power to others).*

4. *Grief - 75: Although they're not as low in boundless energy as someone who is apathetic, someone at the level of grief feels generally depressed about life, and often has a tragic view of the world, accompanied by feelings of regret and sadness.*

5. *Fear - 100: Someone operating at this level has anxiety, paranoia, fear of rejection, fear of failure, fear of uncertainty, fear of challenges, fear of aging, fear of death, fear of loss, fear of strangers, and an overall sense that the world is a scary and frightening place.*

6. *Desire - 125: At this "grass is always greener on the other side" level, one has constant cravings for more money, a better life, better sex, and hedonistic consumption of goods and pursuit of pleasures. This can lead to a never-ending loop of consumption and dissatisfaction. On a positive note, this and future stages are at least those in which someone is taking actions and attempting to move forward and make progress in life.*

7. *Anger - 150: This level is associated with hate, resentment, frustration, toxicity and revenge (think of an Internet troll), often manifesting in irritable behavior, arguments and aggression.*

8. *Pride - 175: Narcissism, ego inflation and scorn or judgment of others dominate at this level, along with a demanding personality and overall arrogance.*

9. *Courage - 200: At this level, one becomes constructive rather than destructive, with a view of the world as exciting and full of possibility, and positive growth if*

one recognizes that they can choose to be happy no matter what the circumstances.

10. Neutrality - 250: At this level, one becomes non-judgmental, objective, and able to begin to see things as they truly are, without excessive attachment to possessions and results, and an ability to be able to adapt to curveballs that life may throw. Occasionally, excessive detachment and carelessness can be issues at this level.

11. Willingness - 310: A high amount of optimism occurs here and, because life is full of hope and meaning, you become full of positive action and open to do anything and everything it takes to succeed.

12. Acceptance - 350: Forgiveness becomes a dominant emotion, and one begins to become more harmonious with themselves and the rest of the world, aware of limiting beliefs and thought patterns.

13. Reason - 400: Understanding, rationality, logic and patient decision-making dominate here, although they are often accompanied by over-intellectualization and an excessive obsession over data.

14. Love - 500: Characterized by pure happiness and goodwill towards others - with a willingness to sacrifice and love fellow humans with no judgment.

15. Joy - 540: The dominant emotions at this level are compassion, happiness, patience, serenity, and a positive attitude. One has not only fully realized that they can choose to be happy no matter the circumstances, but they actually are happy.

16. Peace - 600: Peace, which I also describe as the absolute and ruthless elimination of haste, hurry, and negative stress in one's life, is a state in which the dominant emotion is bliss and pure satisfaction.

17. Enlightenment - 700-1000: This ultimate pinnacle of emotion is often associated with fully enlightened consciousness, and conscientious figures in history such as Krishna, Buddha, and Jesus.

Like Lipton, Hawkins teaches that illness tends to result from suppressed and repressed negative emotions (especially those emotions associated with the lower levels of consciousness you've just read about), followed by a thought that gives that emotion a specific form. A thought has energy and form, and the mind with its thoughts and feelings controls the body. Therefore, to heal the body from the inside-out, thoughts and feelings need to be changed, because what is held in mind tends to express itself through the body, which is like a puppet controlled by the mind. Thoughts are caused by suppressed and repressed feelings, but when a feeling is let go, thousands or even millions of thoughts that were activated by that feeling disappear. You surrender a feeling by allowing it to be there without condemning, judging, or resisting it. Instead, you simply look at it, observe it, and allow it to be felt without trying to modify it.

Hawkins emphasizes that it is important to understand that feelings are not the real self. Whereas feelings are programs that come and go, the real inner self always stays the same—therefore, it is necessary to stop identifying transient feelings as yourself. No matter what is going on in life, keep the steadfast intention to surrender negative feelings as they arise. Make a decision that freedom is more desirable than having a negative feeling, and choose to surrender negative feelings rather than express them, while also surrendering resistance to and skepticism about positive feelings.

In addition, especially when focused on fixing an illness or injury, or keeping one from happening in the first place, associate with people who are using the same or similar motivation and who have the intention to express these positive feelings and to heal. Be aware that your inner state is known and transmitted. The people around you will intuit - based on your electromagnetic signals from your heart and your brain, along with your overall vibrational frequency - what you are feeling and thinking, even if you don't vocally verbalize it.

How Your Environment & Emotions Impact Your Genes & Your Health

The field of research into microRNA reveals that our guts and genes can also have an impact on our personality, emotions, and character. These microRNA, which are small RNA molecules found in plants, animals, and some viruses, are tiny trafficking proteins that modify the behavior of our genes. A single human gene can make over 200 different proteins depending on its microRNA and environment. Your capacity to regenerate organs and to "build a new body every day" is highly dependent on these microRNA.

If you do the math, with your approximately 20,000 genes, you can create somewhere around 4 million different bodies today. If you've built a positive emotional and physical environment and ecosystem around yourself that's allowing you to build that body, this means you have almost incalculable capacity to change who and how you feel today by changing the environment around you. But if you have a chronic ailment—whether it's something as minor as postnasal drainage and chronic congestion or diarrhea, constipation, chronic bloating, obesity, or even depressive thought patterns or negative people around you—then your microRNA become capable of creating a body that comprised of broken components.

These microRNA, derived from the non-coding or non-gene regions of your DNA, can leave the cell and even leave your body. For example, right now, if a physician was to swab your mouth, they could extract microRNA clusters that are in your saliva, and if they go and analyze these microRNA, they can tell exactly what genes you're starting to turn on and off. These microRNA can also be analyzed in urine, breath, and sweat. This means you have tiny packets of data going out into the environment around you. If you sit in a lecture hall, over the course of an hour, the professor could slightly change everybody's genome in the room by exhaling their microRNA into the room, and the trees, the soil, and the fungi in the environment you live in are performing the same actions with their own microRNA. In addition, the bacteria in your gut are making at least 35% of the microRNA that winds up in your bloodstream, and is then sweated out, breathed out, urinated out (or salivated out into the body of another person when you kiss them!). This means that not only are your genes heavily influenced by other people and the environment you're living in, but 35% of what you're giving out to the world is technically nonhuman and made by the bacteria inside you. Many studies have also suggested that how we think and feel are controlled by these microRNA.

Another example of the interplay between biology and consciousness can be seen in the realm of cannabinoids, which are derivatives that are either compounds occurring naturally in the plant Cannabis Sativa. For example, the first and most widely investigated of all the cannabinoids is Δ9-tetrahydrocannabinol (Δ9-THC), which is the main psychotropic constituent of cannabis and the one that undergoes significant binding to cannabinoid receptors in your body—most notably CB1 and CB2 receptors. Two very similar endogenous cannabinoids are anandamide and 2-arachidonoylglycerol (2-AG). Over the years, a significant number of articles have been published in the field of endogenous cannabinoids and have shown that the endocannabinoid system controls multiple functions involving consciousness, including feeding, pain, learning, memory, pain perception, emotions, sleep-wake cycles, and dreaming.

So sometimes working on your spiritual health, especially in matters of emotion or consciousness, involves simultaneously working on your biological health—and also considering the biological and emotional health of those you surround yourself with! In summary, there's a big positive emotional and physical payoff to surrounding yourself with positive people, being positive yourself, and being cognizant of your own internal microbiome and the amount of time you spend in nature surrounded by a natural, flourishing microbiome.

In summary, to begin to heal your body with your mind, you must understand that you are only subject to what you hold in mind. You are only subject to a negative thought or belief if you consciously or unconsciously say that it applies to you. Just imagine the vast array of possibilities that exist once you begin to implement these principles. If you think you are tired, you can become tired. If you think you are sick, you can become sick. If you think you are bold and courageous, you can become bold and courageous. If you think you are happy, you can become a more joyful person to be around. You get the idea.

WHAT THE BIBLE SAYS ABOUT BONE HEALTH (& OVERALL SOUNDNESS OF BODY)

Despite me respecting and finding a great deal of insight and wisdom from the work of many I've cited in this article, including Bruce Lipton, David Hawkins, and Amit Goswami, my source of absolute truth is always the Bible; and with increasing frequency, I turn to the Scriptures over and over again to see whether the work of philosophers and physicians like those I've described above is actually backed up by the Word of God.

And I'm always pleasantly surprised by what I find.

Consider the words of Isaiah 58:10-11, a passage I recently stumbled upon that draws a fascinating corollary between charity, empathy, and service for the needy and bone density (admittedly, in Hebrew literature, bone health is also indicative of overall soundness of flesh and body, and overall mortality - and in Chinese medicine, presence or absence of cancers):

"If you pour yourself out for the hungry and satisfy the desire of the afflicted, then shall your light rise in the darkness and your gloom be as the noonday. And the Lord will guide you continually and satisfy your desire in scorched places and make your bones strong; and you shall be like a watered garden, like a spring of water, whose waters do not fail."

The relationship between state of the mind, state of the emotions, and bones, in particular, is also emphasized in the following verses from the Bible:

Psalms 32:3-5: *"When I kept silent, my bones wasted away through my groaning all day long. For day and night your hand was heavy on me; my strength was sapped as in the heat of summer. Then I acknowledged my sin to you and did not cover up my inequity. I said, 'I will confess my transgressions to the Lord.' And you forgave the guilt of my sin."*

Proverbs 14:30: *"A peaceful heart is life to the body, but envy rots the bones."*

Proverbs 15:30: *"Light in a messenger's eyes brings joy to the heart, and good news gives health to the bones."*

Proverbs 12:4: *"A wife of noble character is her husband's crown, but she who causes shame is like decay in his bones."*

Proverbs 17:22: *"A merry heart does good like a medicine: but a broken spirit dries the bones."*

Proverbs 3:7-8: *"Do not be wise in your own eyes; fear the Lord and turn away from evil. This will bring healing to your body and refreshment to your bones."*

What repeated themes do you see here?

I personally see the following factors all being cited as detrimental to the overall soundness of flesh and bones:

- *Hidden sin, guilt, or bitterness stowed away in one's heart...*

- *Excessive stress, and the absence of peace...*

- *Relationships that are associated with emotions of shame or strife...*

- *A lack of joy and happiness...*

- *An absence of humility, paired with an oversized ego...*

So one could, therefore, say that when it boils down to what the Bible tells us about our health—particularly our bones—that love, humility, and transparency in relationships, a focus on freedom from suppressed anger or bitterness, low amounts of chronic stress accompanied by a trust in God, and seeking sources of joy and happiness (children, hobbies, art, music, funny movies and most importantly, supreme satisfaction in God and his creation) all seem to have a profound impact on health, backing up once again the importance of a sound spirit, a sound body, and a sound mind.

SUMMARY

So when it comes to cancer, bone density, mortality, and overall soundness of body and mind, you can see that Doron became peaceful by shifting himself from the oh-so-typical Western competitive go-go-go lifestyle to an environment of peace and stillness.

Chinese Traditional Medicine has known for thousands of years that worry, fear, hesitation, anger, irritation, nervousness, and the like should all be prevented to maximize health.

Bruce Lipton, David Hawkins, Amit Goswami, and a host of additional authors, researchers, and physicians have demonstrated the intimate link between our state-of-mind, emotions, and biology.

And finally, the Bible backs all of this up, once again clearly demonstrating that you can't Crossfit, triathlon-ercize, or vegan, Carnivore and keto diet your way into ultimate health, nor can you simply take calcium pills for bone density or chemo, fasting and vitamin C IV's for cancer.

That's all I have for you today.

But if you want more, then read Chapters 15, 19, 20, and 21 of my book *"Boundless"*, in which I teach you how to use potent tactics such as purpose, gratitude, prayer, yoga, breathwork, visualization, mindfulness meditation, tapping, acupuncture, sound healing, and many other modalities to improve immunity, lifespan, and health. In the meantime, I encourage you to consider how you care for your own emotional and spiritual health and pay attention to what you experienced as a health or biological result from those practices. The two factors are more intertwined than most people suspect! Finally, how do you know if all of these spiritual fitness and emotional health practices are actually "working" on your physical body? The next chapter will answer that very question.

For resources, references, links and additional reading and listening material for this chapter, visit FitSoulBook.com/Chapter15.

CHAPTER XVI

HOW TO LISTEN TO YOUR BODY

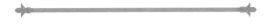

Your body is intelligent.

It sends you subtle messages and cues about your state of stress and readiness that—if you learn to listen—can save you from injury, illness, and even chronic disease.

As Sayer Ji writes in his book *Regenerate* and Jeffrey Rediger in *Cured: The Life-Changing Science of Spontaneous Healing,* **your** body can, when immersed in the correct nourishing and loving environment, repair and renew itself—very much *unlike* a car, which would never spontaneously repair a dent, faulty wiring, or worn brake pad.

By tuning in to and listening to the messages your body sends you each day—whether regarding fitness, food, relationships, or business decisions—you can enhance your ability to be an expert pilot of the finely tuned and intricately designed craft that is your human form.

On the contrary, if you rely purely upon self-quantifying wearable devices and take an all-too-popular modern biohacking and data-driven approach to "listening" to the body, you can often miss those subtle cues from your body and ironically, grow more *distant* from being able to care for yourself as intelligently as you could.

Anyone who relies upon a sleep device such as WHOOP, Oura, DREEM, or Biostrap for self-quantification knows exactly what I mean. You may wake well-rested, refreshed, and energized from what you thought was an amazing night of sleep, but upon glancing at your wearable metrics, you're suddenly confronted with a screen that warns you that your deep sleep was 10% lower than usual and that you had an abnormally high nighttime heart rate, thus your "readiness" for the day is supposedly quite low.

Bubble burst, right?

The placebo effect of being told by a computer that you're not rested can fill you with a sense of stress and unrest and influences you to make a decision to put the brakes on anything mildly stressful or meaningfully productive for the day, causing you instead to choose to take a long nap, skip a meeting, or forego a workout.

Of course, the opposite is also true.

You may wake with a sore and tired body, craving a cup of strong coffee and feeling as though you barely slept a wink, but when you glance at your sleep app feedback, it shows you a giant "thumbs up" with a congratulatory gold star for sleep, and tells you to go crush the day. So you venture forth, push through tiredness, and experience a somewhat unproductive and unpleasant day as you fight through fatigue because, well, your *computer* told you you were just fine.

What a conundrum!

After all, as any regular reader of some of my more edgy scientific fitness or recovery content knows, I'm certainly not *against* self-quantification, wearables, and informed feedback from the impressive variety of devices that can easily track body temperature, heart rate, heart rate variability, respiratory rate, sleep cycles and a host of other metrics—metrics that can often, with laser-like precision, inform you as to the general status of your physiological state.

Yet, constant plugged-in reliance upon these devices as the sole source of your decision making about training, recovery, business, food, and more can ironically distance you from the ability to be able to pay attention to and develop an intimate relationship with the innate intelligence God built in to your body and the signals it is sending you.

So how do you know?

How do you know if that mental resistance to go work out is you just being lazy, or a true sign that you shouldn't train or should opt for something more restorative like yoga or sauna?

How do you know if that dread of placing a heavy barbell on your shoulders for a back squat is because your body doesn't need the chaos, damage, or overtraining that might create on an anatomical or physiological level, or whether your body is instead resisting discomfort and the orderliness, strength, and stability that hard squat day might create for you?

How do you know if you're craving carbs due to an addiction to sugar or the need for a quick dopamine hit or to drown feelings of bitterness and remorse, or whether your body is actually asking you for a much-needed refill of liver or muscle glycogen stores?

How do you know if you truly need more sleep, or if you're just avoiding a tough workday, you're depressed, or you're procrastinating in bed?

How do you know if you desire that glass of wine as a palate cleanser and an enjoyable part of a well-balanced meal or if you want that hit on a vape pen for a whiff of the flavor and relaxing properties of the cannabis plant, or if you're numbing pain and escaping via an exogenous substance?

While self-quantification metrics can certainly *help* in these situations, they can't identify feelings such as pain, depression, laziness, and anger; and they can also remove you from being able to truly listen to your body and understand in a deeper,more intuitive and ancestral way what your body is really trying to tell you.

This in and of itself is quite ironic, because this fascinating and complex interweb of flesh, fascia, blood, and bones is what houses your spirit and soul and enables you to live your very purpose—yet, like a cyclist who can't change a flat tire or an airline pilot who doesn't know how to read the cockpit instrumentation, you often have no clue about your state of health because you simply haven't come to know your body and listen to your body without the help of technology.

So how do you listen to your body?

Embrace stillness.

Embrace silence.

When you wake, spend a few extra moments in bed breathing, wiggling your toes, wiggling your fingers, and tuning into your body. Before a workout or any other stressful event, take a deep centering breath in through your nose, then out through slightly pursed lips. Before you grab a handful of almonds or a cup of coffee or a chunk of dark chocolate, pause and take a few more deep breaths—are you truly hungry, or thirsty, or are you simply drowning yourself with a temporary caloric distraction?

Throughout the day, continue this habit: Step away from the computer, turn off the podcasts, audiobooks, music, and all the background noise and simply ask your body,

"How are you?". Then, be still for several seconds and listen to the subtle internal, intuitive cues of your heart rate, your muscle tension, your gut fullness, and your breath rate.

In other words, be as fully present as you can at all times. Read Chapter 2 if you don't know how to do that. Ultimately, you'll become better at picking up on the subtle clues your body is sending you throughout the day, and more intimately familiar with your body, which is all-so-easy to lose a deep intimate connection with.

Then, sure, use your fancy self-quantification devices and wearables, but marry that modern science to ancestral wisdom. Don't completely outsource everything to a computer. Learn to step away from the chaos, the numbers, the apps, and the screens into the still, small silence, and listen to your body.

For more, I highly recommend you read Chapter 13 about mindful and grateful eating, listen to my podcast (linked to on the resources page for his chapter) with Paul Chek about intuitive eating, and also read the excellent book The Yoga of Eating: Transcending Diets and Dogma to Nourish the Natural Self by Charles Eisenstein.

How about you? Are you married to metrics? Or do you know how to listen to your body, too? In my opinion, there's no better time of day to practice listening to your body than just before you lay your head to sleep in the quiet of the night. Do you have difficulty relaxing, shutting down, sleeping or staying asleep at night? Then by all means, keep reading.

For resources, references, links and additional reading and listening material for this chapter, visit FitSoulBook.com/Chapter16.

CHAPTER XVII

Now I Lay Me Down to Sleep

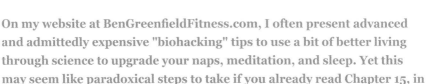

On my website at BenGreenfieldFitness.com, I often present advanced and admittedly expensive "biohacking" tips to use a bit of better living through science to upgrade your naps, meditation, and sleep. Yet this may seem like paradoxical steps to take if you already read Chapter 15, in which I present a stripped-down, minimalist approach to eschewing excessive reliance upon science and self-quantification and instead learning how to intuitively listen to one's body.

So I thought that in this chapter I would revisit the concept of optimizing your sleep and rest, and to specifically highlight that fact that I do not think you necessarily need to stick laser lights up your nose, swallow a cattle trough's worth of supplement capsules, and sleep on a special mat you had to mortgage your house to afford in order to wake up refreshed the next morning.

As a matter of fact, the foundational principles of getting a good night's sleep—no matter your biohacking or healthy living budget—are largely based upon five key spiritual and psychological principles that anyone can implement. Basic concepts of sleep hygiene set aside (which I outline in great detail in my book Boundless), the five key principles to get better sleep naturally are as follows:

1) Relax

You *must* activate your parasympathetic, rest-and-digest nervous system prior to rest. Even seemingly "restful" activities, such as ensuring you have a full stomach and/or drinking a few relaxing glasses of wine, will temporarily make you sleepy; but once those wear off (typically around 1 or 2 am), your body can be flooded with a rebound rush of hypoglycemia and excitatory neurotransmitters. Even ancient writers of Scriptures knew this. Consider verses such as:

Ecclesiastes 5:12: *"Sweet is the sleep of a laborer, whether he eats little or much, but the full stomach of the rich will not let him sleep."*

1 Thessalonians 5:7: *"For those who sleep, sleep at night, and those who get drunk, are drunk at night."*

So, figure out how to relax your body and brain prior to sleep! Supplements and biohacks aside (as will be the theme of this chapter), you can try a series of simple yoga moves like those that I'll link to on the resources page for this chapter, moves that you can perform by your bedside, accompanied by deep, nasal breathing. You can keep the lights dim, switch to incandescent red bulbs instead of flourescent or LED lighting, or even adopt the use of nighttime candles in your bedroom. You can finish any hard workouts 3 hours before bed to keep the body's core temperature low or, as my friend Hylke Reitsma wrote in a recent guest post on my own website, you can adopt a "10-3-2-1-0 sleep routine":

- *10 - The number of hours before sleep in which you do not consume caffeine*

- *3 - The number of hours before sleep in which you do not eat (or drink, but that is up for debate)*

- *2 - The number of hours before sleep in which you do not work*

- *1 - The number of hours before sleep in which you do not engage in screen time*

- *0 - The number of times you hit the snooze button*

2) Read

Once you are relaxed, crawl into bed and grab a bedside book that isn't about topics that get you excited, such as fitness or business, but instead are relaxing, philosophical or fictional reads that charm your mind with positive, affirmative thoughts prior to bed. Ideally, these books should not be consumed on a Kindle, smartphone, or any other e-reader due to the presence of light that can shut down your natural melatonin product, but rather in paper form. For example, a few of the books I'm reading right now for bedtime include *The Way To Love* by Anthony De Mello, *Orthodoxy* by G.K. Chesterton, *Ride, Sally, Ride* by Doug Wilson and *Desiring God* by John Piper.

3) Meditate or Pray

My favorite app for bedtime meditation is Abide, a Christian app chock-full of sleep-enhancing and deeply relaxing and restorative nighttime stories and meditations (admittedly, I believe this, and the books I cite above, are the only somewhat "non-free" items on my list.) Another very good one for those who are religiously and spiritually inclined is the free app Pause. However, I often simply close my eyes, and, along with my wife—with whom I keep a bedside list of family members, friends, and topics to bring to the Lord—utter a few simple prayers of gratitude, praise, and supplication to God. If there is any sin harbored in my heart, especially anger or feelings of unrest towards any people in my life, I bring those feelings to the Lord in a spirit of confession and repentance, heeding the words of Ephesians 4:26, which reads:

> *"Be angry and do not sin; do not let the sun go down on your anger."*

If you're not accustomed to praying prior to falling asleep, or don't know where to start, try the relatively well-known verses below. Although their origin is obscure, you'll find them quite settling to your spirit in times of stress or insomnia:

> *"Now I lay me down to sleep.*
> *I pray the Lord my soul to keep.*
> *If I should die before I wake,*
> *I pray to God my soul to take.*
> *If I should live for other days,*
> *I pray the Lord to guide my ways.*
> *Father, unto thee I pray,*
> *Thou hast guarded me all day;*
> *Safe I am while in thy sight,*
> *Safely let me sleep tonight.*
> *Bless my friends, the whole world bless;*
> *Help me to learn helpfulness;*
>
> *Keep me every in thy sight;*
> *So to all I say good night."*

4) Breathe

While there are a multitude of forms of relaxing breathwork, many of which I discuss in great detail in my book Boundless, two of my favorites are a "double-inhale-to-exhale" and a "4-7-8" pattern. For the former, my friend and brilliant neuroscientist, Dr. Andrew Huberman, who I first mentioned in Chapter 12, claims that breaking up one long inhale as a double inhale through your nose and then exhaling through your mouth can calm you instantly. It seems to work. My friend Dr. Andrew Weil favors the 4-7-8 protocol, and this one also seems to work quite well. Relying upon your own breath is, of course, the last time I checked, also free.

5) Trust

Fall asleep with a smile on your face, trusting God that he will provide for tomorrow.

Matthew 6:25-27 tells us:

> *"Therefore I tell you, do not worry about your life, what you will eat or drink; or about your body, what you will wear. Is not life more than food, and the body more than clothes? Look at the birds of the air: They do not sow or reap or gather into barns— and yet your Heavenly Father feeds them. Are you not much more valuable than they? Who of you by worrying can add a single hour to his life?"*

Psalm 4:8 says:

> *"In peace I will both lie down and sleep; for you alone, O Lord, make me dwell in safety." and Psalm 91:1-16: "He who dwells in the shelter of the Most High will abide in the shadow of the Almighty. I will say to the Lord, "My refuge and my fortress, my God, in whom I trust." For he will deliver you from the snare of the fowler and from the deadly pestilence. He will cover you with his pinions, and under his wings you will find refuge; his faithfulness is a shield and buckler. You will not fear the terror of the night, nor the arrow that flies by day". Finally, when it comes to the spirit of bringing any of your burdens to the great heavenly Father, nothing is quite as clear as Matthew 11:28, which reads: "Come to me, all who labor and are heavy laden, and I will give you rest."*

Now don't get me wrong: I'm not the spiritually enlightened yet lazy fellow who simply trusts God then sits back, laces my hand behind my head and stares at the sky while laying in a hammock all day and waiting for God to provide. Rather, I'm a firm believer that one should trust God, then "put on their seatbelt", as the saying goes. Or perhaps more Biblically appropriate is the approach in Nehemiah 4:9, which states *"...we prayed to our God and posted a guard day and night to meet this threat.".*

In other words, cast your cares upon God when you can't get to sleep at night or you wake up with racing thoughts, but don't completely ignore or discount thoughts, ideas or insight God gives you as you're falling asleep or waking in the wee hours. My own strategy for this is to keep a simple Pilot pen light and paper journal next to my bed at night so I can (without needing to grab my phone, which is a major mistake when attempting to optimize sleep) jot anything down that I need to, get it "out of my head", then fall back asleep.

Summary

So sleep really can be that simple, my friends.

Can't stomach supplements?

Don't want to fork over the cash for fancy biohacks?

Resisted to feeling as though you may become "attached" to a host of items that you rely upon for sleep?

Then use these easy, inexpensive, spiritual, and psychological sleep and relaxation methods—*relax, read, pray, breathe, and trust*—the next time you're tossing and turning, or crave a good night's sleep, and you'll be pleasantly surprised at the results.

I encourage you to turn to these simple tools before launching into all the "fancy stuff" constantly championed and marketed for sleep improvement. I suspect you'll be surprised at how simple sleep can be, especially when you place your trust in the Almighty Creator. If you like the idea of simplicity, yet find yourself constantly pulled into the more advanced and confusing world of self-quantification and metric tracking (something all-too-commonly relied upon in the health and fitness world) then you'll discover in the next chapter how to simplify that approach too.

For resources, references, links and additional reading and listening material for this chapter, visit FitSoulBook.com/Chapter17.

CHAPTER XVIII

HOPE

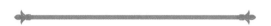

Ah, how complex is the ever-evolving science of self-quantification!

In Chapter 15, I tackled the world of wearables—and the importance of knowing how to unplug from our rings, wristbands, ankle bracelets, chips, watches, and miniature body computers to instead listen to the oh-so-subtle cues from our body and it's innate intelligence.

But beyond these computerized devices is an entirely different realm: that softer science of blood and biomarker testing. I've exhaustively tackled this topic in the past in my book *Boundless* and in a host of articles I'll link to on the resources page for this chapter, highlighting the importance—should you be concerned about your overall health and longevity—of tracking variables such as inflammation, glycemic variability, hormones, lipids, ketones, genes, the microbiome, and more.

Yet, of all the varying and ever-expanding forms of self-quantification that exist, there is one single asset you can possess that is far more crucial to your overall health and longevity than your HDL, your testosterone, your ketone levels, your step count, your grip strength, or any other quantifiable variable...

...hope.

THE IMPORTANCE OF HOPE

In secular psychology, hope is defined as a motivation to persevere toward a goal or end state, even when you may be skeptical that a positive outcome is likely.

It often involves proactive progress toward a goal, a can-do attitude, and a belief that you have some kind of achievable pathway to a desired outcome.

But as a Christian, I tend to lean towards preferring pastor and author John Piper's definition of hope just a bit better than that above. Piper says...

..."Hope is a heartfelt, joyful conviction that our short-term future is governed by an all-caring God, and our long-term future, beyond death, will be happy beyond imagination in the presence of the all-satisfying glory of God."

How much more meaningful (and hopeful!) life can be when we believe that our story has a great Author, rather than believing that everything we see and experience is meaningless and without purpose, or that we are simply a bunch of chunks of spiritless flesh and blood floating through space on a giant rock, then eventually dying and passing away into nothingness.

It turns out that, very similar to what we know about the human science of a gratitude practice, and what we know about the power of having a purpose statement in life, the physical and psychological impact of the emotion of hope is also quite impressive.

For example, one study from Harvard's "Human Flourishing Program" examined the impact of hope on nearly 13,000 people and found those with more hope in their lives had superior physical health, better overall health behaviors, increased social support, and a longer life—along with fewer chronic health problems, less depression and anxiety, and a lower risk of cancer. Long-term studies of employee well-being suggest that hopeful employees experience more well-being, and in one Gallup poll of 1 million students, those who were more hopeful laughed and smiled much more often than the hopeless, and also engaged in healthier behaviors, including fruit and vegetable consumption, regular exercise, safer sex practices, and less smoking. In his book, *The Anatomy Of Hope*, Dr. Jerome Groopman, Professor and Chairman of the Department of Medicine at Harvard Medical School, tells extraordinary stories of hope in coping with conventionally hopeless diseases and suffering. He demonstrates that on a biological level, hope may stimulate the release of internal painkiller molecules.

Hope not only changes us physically, but also psychologically. Hope empowers us to endure greater amounts of suffering. In times of crisis or survival, even a small glimpse of hope can infuse greater endurance and strength into our circumstances. It produces opportunity and proactiveness, because when you live with the expectation that positive changes are on the horizon, you can open yourself up to a world of new possibilities, fueled by confidence that a new way of life is possible rather than being paralyzed by fear of an unknown, dark and scary future. Hope brings forth purpose and vision, infuses joy and happiness, and gives us a glimpse in our weary lives that, as the famous Christmas song O Holy Night goes, yonder breaks a new and glorious morn:

> *"Long lay the world in sin and error pining,*
> *Till He appear'd and the soul felt its worth.*
> *A thrill of hope, the weary world rejoices,*
> *For yonder breaks a new and glorious morn."*

One could argue that the opposite of hope is helplessness. For example, in a series of 1965 experiments that you're likely familiar with, researcher Martin Seligman discovered learned helplessness when he observed that animals subjected to difficult situations they cannot control will stop trying to escape, and instead become submissive and passive. Here's an illustration of one such example of dogs in an electrified cage:

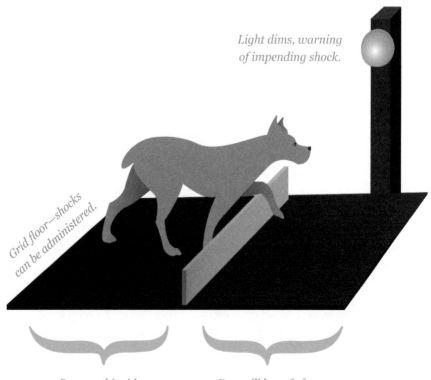

Light dims, warning of impending shock.

Grid floor—shocks can be administered.

Bars on this side will be electrified.

Dog will be safe from shock on this side.

In summary:

- *Dogs are in an electrified cage at first not able to escape the impending shock.*

- *Later, all they had to do was cross to the other side to escape the shock, but they didn't even try.*

- *The dogs had learned they were "helpless" to avoid the shock and so they just sat there and took the shock without trying to escape.*

Human beings are the same. If we experience devastating defeats, a persistent situation that we can't change, or a terrifying event that we cannot control our exposure to, we can often lose hope for our ability to change this painful situation. Apathy sets in. We don't try to get a job, make friends, eat healthier, leave a partner who may be abusive, or engage in other efforts to proactively make life better. We tend to see *any* efforts to change our life as largely futile. We accept whatever happens as beyond our control. We begin to despair.

After all, why bother? It won't really make a difference. We don't want to risk the pain of further disappointment by even trying. Unfortunately, this despair and resignation can become a self-fulfilling negative cycle. If you have no hope that any action you take will make any difference, then that often very well is the actual outcome.

So let me ask you, which would you rather have: hope or helplessness?

THE IMPORTANCE OF HOPE

Now that you understand the immense importance of waking up each day with not only a strong sense of purpose and gratitude, but also a deep sense of hope, how can you best tap into this powerful emotion?

Here are a few good tips for discovering more hope, particularly when you're in a bit of a funk or feeling down:

-*Consider all the amazing things you've done in your life.* In other words, remember past positive experiences, which I would consider to tie closely to a daily practice of gratitude, or at least to be far easier when you're able to crack open the pages of a gratitude journal and see what you've written on previous days.

-Surround yourself with optimism. Try to hang out with people who persistently see the bright side of things and the sunny side of every situation—who always have a smile and a positive attitude.

-Surround yourself with inspiration. Pipe uplifting music into your home, allow sun to constantly be seeping in through the windows, engage in exposure to fresh air and nature immersion, seep yourself with aromatherapy via uplifting scents such as peppermint, rose, or cinnamon; and surround yourself with inspirational memes, quotes, and artwork on your walls and screensavers. You'd be surprised at how simple environmental tweaks can produce a near-instant positive impact on mode.

-Write down a plan. If there are changes that need to be made in your life, such as a new workout plan to get through an injury, a new weekly schedule to free up time for a project you've been neglecting, or a book-reading schedule to get through a new series you've been wanting to read, then you must understand that being able to see how the steps you are taking will lead to desired change is critical to producing hope. Write down each step that you need to take to get where you want to be.

-Check out ProjectHopeExchange.com. This is a website where people record their experiences of overcoming adversity, and there is a special section for mental health challenges and life challenges. It turns out there are many people who have overcome tremendous adversity. Reading their stories and surrounding yourself with the supportive messages you'll find there can help you build hope.

-Take every step you can. Do what you know you can do. When you are in despair, taking one tiny step forward can help break any sense of hopelessness you may have. Feeling depressed or hopeless about the day? Make your bed. Cook breakfast. Meditate for five minutes. Call a friend. Take the small steps you know you can take. One common piece of wisdom in wilderness survival, and a common trait in those who survive through very difficult survival conditions, is that they are constantly taking tiny steps to make their situation just a little bit better—no matter how small those steps may be.

-Help others. Performing acts of kindness can have a dramatic effect on your mood and outlook. Kindness triggers the release of serotonin, so it can produce an anti-depressant effect; and, similar to what you'll experience with a gratitude practice, an increased sense of empathy in your own life can help to calm stress, reduce pain and increase hope.

-Finally, the biggest tip that I can give you for finding hope is to embrace faith and

to engage with a religious or spiritual community. Since the dawn of time, it has repeatedly been shown that when surrounded by a community of like-minded and supportive believers, people have drawn strength, found peace, and experienced an overall elevation of positive well being, fueled by the hope of knowing there is something or someone much larger than them, watching over and protecting them along each step of life's winding path.

While many would scoff at the belief that there are gods and demons, spirits and angels, and even one single almighty Creator of the planet, research has indeed shown a connection between longevity and faith. One study entitled *Church Attendance, Allostatic Load and Mortality in Middle-Aged Adults* analyzed the relationship between religious practice, stress, and death in middle age, and controlled for socioeconomic factors, health insurance status, and healthy lifestyle behaviors. The researchers found that churchgoers have a significantly lower risk of dying, and after adjusting for age, sex, race, and chronic medical conditions, churchgoers were 46% less likely to die in the follow-up period after the study compared to non-churchgoers. Non-churchgoers had significantly higher rates of blood pressure and a higher ratio of total cholesterol to HDL cholesterol, along with a significantly higher mortality rate.

It turns out that data from *The Blue Zones* — areas with a disproportionately high number of healthy, so-called "centenarians"—backs this up. All but five of the 263 centenarians that author Dan Buettner interviewed for the book belonged to some faith-based community. Research also shows that attending faith-based services four times per month can add four to fourteen years of life expectancy. In all Blue Zones, centenarians were part of a religious community. I can't sum it up any better than Buettner, who concluded that:

"People who pay attention to their spiritual side have lower rates of cardiovascular disease, depression, stress, and suicide, and their immune systems seem to work better ... To a certain extent, adherence to a religion allows them to relinquish the stresses of everyday life to a higher power."

In the Bible, which is of course a perfect example of a highly valued source of absolute truth for many faith-based communities, 1 Peter 5:7 recommends us to *"cast all our cares upon Him."* Being able to "cast my cares" and to be able to trust in and talk to a higher power, buttressed by the support and encouragement of others who are also believers, is certainly something that has given me personally a great deal of hope, confidence, clarity, peace, and direction in life. When it comes to your own health, I am convinced that a religious practice that includes spiritual disciplines such as fasting, meditation, prayer, silence, solitude, worship, and study is magnitudes more meaningful and impactful than a salad of herbs and wild plants, a glass of organic wine, or a megadose of sunshine and fresh air.

Of course, this entire faith, healing, and hope trilogy is all supported to the underlying science behind the biology of belief and impact of emotional state on your flesh and bones that I teach you about in Chapter 14. To discover this hope, read about the Hero's Journey in Chapter 9 and begin to understand the vast significance of being able to, without any sense of shame or judgment, cast every last care and both the lightest and heaviest of burdens upon Him. John Piper describes this flavor of hope as a *"vibrant, living, unshakable, blood-bought hope that is the defining motion of the Christian heart and gives rise to joyful fearlessness in the face of human trouble and threats."*

When you discover a hope that epic in your life, and it's planted like a flourishing, fragrant flower within the garden of your heart, you'll find that every other form of self-quantification pales in terms of being able to "predict" your health and lifespan. Nothing is more important.

Furthermore, if you have already discovered that hope, and you wish to share a defense for the hope that is within you, then I recommend that you read the book *Always Ready: Directions for Defending the Faith* by Greg Bahnsen. This book is an excellent compilation of several of Dr. Bahnsen's published works on Christian apologetics, including his Apologetics syllabus, articles on practical apologetic problems like the problem of evil, the problem of miracles, etc. It will allow you to better share your hope with others who have yet to discover the intense meaning in life derived from a strong sense of hope, and to fulfill the words of 1 Peter 3:15 in the Bible...

> ..."*Always be prepared to give an answer to everyone who asks you to give the reason for the hope that you have.*"

How about you? Do you have hope in your life? If so, how do you feed the fire of hope that is within you? Are you able to share an answer to others about the source of the hope that is within you? In the same way that you can consider hope to be fuel for your spiritual journey, you can consider union with God to be the source of strength for that journey. In the next chapter, I'll teach you how to pair hope with that union.

For resources, references, links and additional reading and listening material for this chapter, visit FitSoulBook.com/Chapter18.

UNION

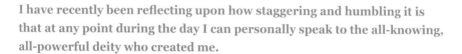

I have recently been reflecting upon how staggering and humbling it is that at any point during the day I can personally speak to the all-knowing, all-powerful deity who created me.

That's a bit of a staggering thought, really.

Just consider for a moment the power, awesomeness, and ultimate greatness of God. Not god, but *God*. Sadly, many do not fully comprehend this greatness.

Allow me to give you two examples.

God is an awesome Being, and I imagine it would be quite paralyzing and terrifying to even look upon Him. In the Bible, Moses, a faithful prophet of God who one would think would certainly be in union with God, was only allowed to see God's back, because otherwise, if he saw God's face he would surely die *("You cannot see My face; for no man shall see Me, and live" - Exodus 33:20)*.

We, like Moses, have little clues about what God actually looks like, but I suspect from the clues that we do have that He is definitely not an old man with a white beard clad in a soft robe sitting on a cloud and strumming a harp. Neither is He a magical, wispy fairy who flitters about sprinkling glitter throughout the universe. In addition, He is surely not what Hollywood portrays Him to be, such as the nice man in a white suit as depicted in Jim Carrey's film Bruce Almighty.

In Isaiah 40:15-17, God says of Himself, *"Behold, the nations are as a drop in a bucket, and are counted as the small dust on the scales; look, He lifts up the isles as a very little thing. And Lebanon is not sufficient to burn, nor its beasts sufficient for a burnt offering. All nations before Him are as nothing, and they are counted by Him less than nothing and worthless."*

God goes on to say in verses 18-19, *"To whom then will you liken God? Or what likeness will you compare to Him? The workman molds an image, the goldsmith overspreads it with gold, and the silversmith casts silver chains."*

In other words, it is impossible for us tiny, feeble humans to fully picture the power and glory of God in our current physical state, nor to fashion or carve any type of image that portrays what He looks like, but it is something altogether mind-blowing. It is beyond our wildest imaginations.

Yet, we often portray God as merely a "special friend," a magical fairy in the sky, or a meek, white-bearded old man.

But God is dangerous. Fierce. Wild. He is a great, roaring lion like the Aslan of Narnia I describe in Chapter 7.

In one article I read several years ago, author Doug Jones portrays a fitting description of God's fierceness, wildness, and dangerousness. He says:

> *"...in our pietism, though, we tend to insist that God is primarily Nice. Period. God is Nice and Nicer and Nicest. The chief end of God is to be Nice. I believe in God the Nice. Maker of Niceness. In heaven, we'll all be Nice. Pilate wasn't Nice. He was mean, and "mean people suck." This whole modern Christian litany is so tedious and tiny. Of course, other people—equally foolish—think the solution is to be rude and mean. Yeah, God isn't nice; He's rude. But Yahweh is neither Nice or Rude: He is dangerous and unpredictable.*

> *He is Trinity. He is Fire, and fire is hard to contain. Sometimes all the advanced firefighting technology gets overcome in a canyon by a storm of flames. Sometimes people freeze next to a tiny flame. Fire's edges won't stand still; its borders aren't easily traced. "Our God is a consuming fire." God's command for Abraham to sacrifice Isaac came right from the center of flame. As H. A. Williams notes, "Whatever God wants in our relationship with Him, it certainly isn't respectability.*

> *"To Moses He was fire. To Ezekiel He wore the symbols of ox, eagle, lion. To Jonah He was a man-eating fish. To Balaam He spoke through donkey lips. Yahweh boasts in animals, especially wild ones. "For every beast of the forest is Mine, and the cattle on a thousand hills. I know all the birds of the mountains, and the wild beasts of the field are Mine" (Ps. 50:10,11).*

The Lord seems to especially love His horses: "Have you given the horse strength? Have you clothed his neck with thunder? He mocks at fear, and is not frightened; nor does he turn back from the sword. He devours the distance with fierceness and rage; nor does he come to a halt because the trumpet has sounded. At the blast of the trumpet he says, `Aha!' He smells the battle from afar" (Job 39:19-25). He loves it that they refuse to stop at the trumpet. What kind of God says that?

Yahweh reveals His dangerousness in hawks and eagles, too. They are His artwork, revealing more of His style: "Does the hawk fly by your wisdom. . . . Does the eagle mount up at your command and make its nest on high? On the rocks it dwells and resides, on the crag of the rock and the stronghold. From there it spies out the prey; its eyes observe from afar. Its young ones suck up blood; and where the slain are, there it is." (Job 39:26-30). The NIV gives, "His young ones feast on blood." But why the detail about blood? Do we really need that? Can't we just talk about porcelain doves? No, God is gloriously dangerous and noble like an eagle. Solomon recognized that "the way of an eagle in the air" is just "too wonderful" (Prov. 30:18,19).

Yahweh reveals Himself in a cheetah kill. Oh, those nice, soft, delicate antelopes. It would be nice to pet them. They should be protected. "Can you hunt the prey for the lion, or satisfy the appetite of the young lions?" (Job 38:39). God can. He's on the run and right in the middle of the lion kill. He boasts in giving them food. He satisfies lions.

Does that mean God hates deer? He's made them just for food? Of course not. He boasts in them, too. "Can you mark when the deer gives birth? Can you number the months that they fulfill? Or do you know the time when they bear young? They bow down, they bring forth their young, they deliver their offspring. Their young ones are healthy, they grow strong with grain; They depart and do not return to them" (Job 39:2-4). He loves them and sometimes loves to feed them to lions. That's the God of Abraham."

A fire, an ox, an eagle, a lion, a man-eating sea monster, a wild stallion, and a soaring

eagle? This certainly doesn't seem like a nice old man in the sky, does it?

Doug goes on to say:

> "...God is dangerous, wild, and unpredictable. He is dynamite and a kidnapper. That's the God of Abraham...the God of Abraham does not pen Hallmark cards. He is not a corporate risk manager. He is not a cruise director aiming to make our trip as pleasant and comfortable as possible. He is here to overturn tables and create people who can run alongside Him. "If you have run with the footmen, and they have wearied you, then how can you contend with horses?" (Jer. 12:5). He wants people like horses, people whose necks are "clothed with thunder," "mock at fear," and do not stop at the sound of the trumpet. It's not about power; it's about character and tension and Trinity.
>
> In the midst of this intricate play of history, tension is normal. Trials and evil are normal. How dare we be surprised by evil? How dare we wish it away, pining for the nursery? That is not the world of the God of Abraham. Williams, again, observes, "Conflict . . . is absolutely necessary if our relationship with God is to grow into maturity. And unless this absolute necessity is recognized, we shall misunderstand what is happening to us and be weighed down by an appalling load of guilt; or we shall press the conflict so that it can find only a sneaking and perverted expression below the level of consciousness while we apparently remain God's good little boys, futile and ineffective half-people."

For some reason beyond our understanding, this wild, fierce and dangerous God also allowed for conflict, turmoil, evils, thorns, thistles, poisonous snakes and spiders, natural disasters, and the like. This does not seem like a Being to ignore, take lightly or take for granted, does it?

So we know that God is wild, fierce, and dangerous, and we also don't know what He looks like. However, and this leads me to my second point, we *can* catch tiny glimpses of God's greatness in the fierce beauty of His Creation.

In Romans 1:20, the apostle Paul states that God's nature, glory, and power are clearly demonstrated in our physical world: *"For since the creation of the world His invisible attributes are clearly seen, being understood by the things that are made, even His eternal power and Godhead..."*

Just think for a moment about the incredible nature of the very planet you walk upon. It is precisely the correct distance from the sun to keep us all from being struck dead by a powerful, burning source of star energy that, in a single second, converts four million tons of matter into pure energy—ninety billion megatons of energy, to be precise.

At the top of our earth's atmosphere is a layer of ozone that filters out most of the harmful ultraviolet light radiated from this sun and allows for a perfect temperature and ratio of gases to sustain life. Additionally, our atmosphere contains a specific and perfectly proportioned ratio of gases that allow life to exist here on earth. Of this sun, and also all its sister stars, David says in Psalm 19:1, *"The heavens declare the glory of God; and the firmament shows His handiwork."*

And how about those stars that go beyond the sun? The number of stars in the universe is unknown, since every time scientists peer deeper into space, they find still more stars. David Kornreich, an astronomer at Ithaca College in New York, gives a rough estimate of 10 trillion galaxies in the universe. Multiplying that by the Milky Way's estimated one hundred billion stars results in approximately 1,000,000,000,000,000,000,000,000 stars, or a one with twenty-four zeros after it (which Kornreich mentions is likely a gross underestimation, as more detailed looks at the universe will show even more galaxies).

Then think beyond the earth, the sun, and the stars and consider the unbelievable complexity of animals. Take an eagle, for example. Job 39:26-29 says: *"Does the hawk fly by your wisdom, and spread its wings toward the south? Does the eagle mount up at your command, and make its nest on high? On the rock it dwells and resides, on the crag of the rock and the stronghold. From there it spies out the prey; its eyes observe from afar."*

It turns out that eagles truly do have incredible eyesight. The eagle eye is among the strongest in the animal kingdom, with an eyesight estimated at 4 to 8 times stronger than that of the average human. An eagle is said to be able to spot a rabbit over two miles away!

Then you can go even tinier than the eye and consider our very cellular enzymes themselves. The more scientists look into cells and enzymes, the more complexity they find. I found a wonderful description of this complexity in the book *"In Six Days,"* where it is described that...

"...only enzymes produce the pure amino acids and sugars necessary for life, but enzyme manufacture requires a living cell. Life is based on life. Then there is the insurmountable problem of getting even one functional enzyme by random processes, even if you could get all the ingredients assembled together. Let us consider just one enzyme comprised of a typical 300 amino acids. Even if we are generous to the materialist and assume that only 150 amino acids have to be specified for the function of the enzyme, the probability of getting a functional sequence is less than 1 in 10. We cannot imagine such an improbability. There are possibly 1080 atoms in the universe. If we made every atom in our universe another universe just like ours, and every one of those atoms were an experiment for every millisecond of the presumed evolutionary age of our universe, this would amount to 10181 experiments – still a long way short of even the remotest chance of getting one functional enzyme. That's just one enzyme. This simplest living cell must have at least several hundred enzymes/proteins..."

You can read more about the complexity of cellular life in articles I will link to on the resources page for this chapter, including *Intelligent Design: Can Science Answer the Question, Does God Exist?, Irreducible Complexity,* **and** *Origin of Life: Are Single Cells Really Simple?*.

This blazing sun, trillions of stars, a protected planet, eagle eyes, cells, and enzymes are obviously just scratching the surface of examples of how God's complexity and greatness shine through in all of creation. Ultimately, God's image and God's creation are spectacular and awe-inspiring. God's dangerous nature is fear-striking and terrifying.

Yet how rarely do we consider the amazing notion that this all-powerful Creator of this entire universe walks among us each day?

How rarely do we consider that we can talk to Him whenever we would like? How more rarely do we actually make any attempt to do so?

Despite being given the privilege of being in union with the greatest being this universe has ever known, most of us spend the majority of our lives disconnected from God, or ignoring the laws He has established for our existence, order, and happiness. These laws, laid out clearly in the greatest book that has ever existed, are not suggestions or tips from a special friend. They are Commandments from our Creator.

I don't know about you, but it gives me pause to consider the grave consequences of ignoring this God, avoiding union with this God, and discounting the wild, fierce, dangerous, complex, mind-blowingly intelligent nature of this God.

Union With God

Yet, magically, this same all-powerful God continues to walk among us mere humans. And, as I alluded to in the introduction to this chapter, we can actually talk to Him. To me, this concept is simultaneously breathtaking and humbling.

Consider the words of Genesis 3:8, which says, *"And they heard the sound of the LORD God walking in the garden in the cool of the day, and the man and his wife hid themselves from the presence of the LORD God among the trees of the garden."* We know that God is spirit (John 4:24), so how exactly could He be "walking" in the garden?

This verse begins by stating, "They heard the *sound*" of God. Whatever form God took when he walked in the garden of Eden, his form somehow allowed for the audible production of sound. The verse also describes the presence of God among the trees of the garden. Do you think God still walks among us? Or do you think that God created this entire complex universe to please Himself and bring Him the greatest glory imaginable, then simply decided to "walk away" and never dwell among us again, instead opting to observe us from a distance while playing a harp on a far-off cloud?

I doubt God has forsaken us. Indeed, I know he has not. As the old gospel song "In The Garden," so beautifully rendered by country artist Merle Haggard here, goes:

> *And he walks with me and he talks with me*
>
> *And he tells me I am his own*
>
> *And the joy we share*
>
> *As we tarry there*
>
> *None other has ever known.*

Yes, God walks among us. He talks to us. We are graciously allowed and privileged to be in union with Him. And—at least for me—that's a pretty humbling and staggering thought to consider.

Three Ways To Maintain Union With God

So don't take for granted the ability to be in daily union with the mightiest King that has ever existed—to walk with Him, talk with Him, and share his joy.

That union is a blessing we all-too-often take for granted.

So I have three simple suggestions for you to maintain your union with God.

First, take everything to God in prayer. He will grant you wisdom and discernment if you ask for it. He will give you answers. All you need do is ask. This week, every day, even with the smallest of decisions, consider coming to God with questions such as "What should I eat?," "Who should I ask about this problem?," "What task should I tackle first?" Then simply stop, breathe, and listen for the still, small voice in the silence. He will give you direction. As you practice listening for the voice of God in silence, consider the words of 1 Kings 19:11-13, which magnify the significance of where God can powerfully speak to us:

> *"Now there was a great wind, so strong that it was splitting mountains and breaking rocks in pieces before the Lord, but the Lord was not in the wind; and after the wind an earthquake, but the Lord was not in the earthquake; and after the earthquake a fire, but*
>
> *the Lord was not in the fire; and after the fire a sound of sheer silence. When Elijah heard it, he wrapped his face in his mantle and went out and stood at the entrance of the cave. Then there came a voice to him that said, "What are you doing here, Elijah?"*

Second, stop at a few points during your busy day, once again breathe, and simply survey the wonders of Creation around you and speak to God a simple phrase: "I am here. Speak to me and show me what You want to teach me." Then, once again, be silent and listen. God's words to you will once again come in the still, small silence. He may ask you to pray. To open a Bible. To call a family member or friend. To step away from work for a moment to meditate or worship. I have personally found the simple "I am here" habit a few times during the day to be a powerful way to stay in union with God.

Third, be grateful and stop to thank God multiple times during the day. In Chapter 12, I told you:

> *"...each night, as I fall asleep to the gentle diaphragmatic lull of my own "4-count-in-8-count-out" breathwork pattern, I'm silently thanking God and trusting God that there will be yet more oxygen available for me for my next inhale. Indeed, the mere act of mindful breathing combined with a silent gratefulness to God for each and every breath is a wonderful practice, and one I recommend you try the next time you're stuck in twenty minutes of traffic. After all, our great Creator smiles when we worship Him, and I certainly think that no king would complain of a subject entering their throne room for several minutes and saying with the deepest gratitude with each breath..."Thank you...thank you...thank you..."*

But don't just thank Him with your breath. Thank Him before a meal. Thank Him when you see a bald eagle soaring overhead. Thank Him when you're stuck in traffic. Thank Him when you get a good email. Thank Him when you get a bad email. Thank Him when a loved one hugs you. Thank Him in *all things*.

Those three simple habits are all it takes to begin your journey into full daily union with God...

..."*What should I do?*"...

..."*I am here.*"...

..."*Thank you.*"

Try it out each week, and I think you'll be amazed and surprised at how God speaks to you when you actually speak to Him, then stop to listen, and as you do so, consider that you are listening to the most wild, fierce, dangerous, complex Being this world has ever known. For more on maintaining this constant, unceasing union with God, I also highly recommend you read the book *"Practicing His Presence"*, a 300 year old book that has never been out of print and that will teach you how to engage in a journey that brings you closer to Christ each day.

SUMMARY

Finally, I'll admit that it can sometimes be difficult to find the time and motivation to stay in the constancy of union with God that you now know is so important. Regarding this, I was recently reading Andrew Murray's provoking book *Absolute Surrender*, in which he says:

> *"The keeping is to be continuous. Every morning, God will meet you as you wake. It is not a question: If I forget to wake in the morning with the thought of Him, what will come of it? If you trust your waking to God, God will meet you in the mornings as you wake with His divine sunshine and life. He will give you the consciousness that through the day you have got God to continually take charge of you with His almighty power. And God will meet you the next day and every day. Never mind if, in the practice of fellowship, failure sometimes comes. If you maintain your position—and say: "Lord, I am going to expect You to do Your utmost, and I am going to trust You day by day to keep me absolutely," your faith will grow stronger and stronger. You will know the keeping power of God in unbrokenness."*

This statement resonated with me: because that daily (specifically morning) keeping of union with God can be hard. I don't know about you, but it's hard for me to wake, suppress the urge to leap from bed and instead actually take the time to breathe, read my Bible, and complete my spiritual disciplines journaling.

It's even *harder* when I'm traveling, and I went to bed later than planned due to late night dinner obligations or had a crappy night of sleep because I'm outside my home environment, and then I wake knowing I'm supposed to be at a conference or meeting in an hour and I have so much to do to get ready, and yet I know that the very *best* thing I can do is greet the day by greeting God.

Heck, even if I set aside for a moment any thoughts of a 10 or 20 minute meditation later in the morning, or squeezing in an AM workout, or having a few quality moments with the family - the mere act of praying, cracking open the Bible, and spending time in God's Word before my feet hit the floor is just *hard*. It takes time. Admittedly, not a ton of time - as ten to fifteen minutes usually suffices for me - but it's time nonetheless.

And it takes trust. Trust that God will provide for me even if I don't bang out those twenty emails that I really want to get off my chest or out of my mind before I start my "real" workday, trust that God will put food on the table even if I don't get those extra precious few minutes of work in, and trust that God will help me remember all those jumbling thoughts marching through my head that I woke up with and I want to act upon right away.

Is it the same for you?

Fortunately, Andrew presents a solution within the pages of the book, and based on the book's title, the solution comes as no surprise: absolute surrender.

He says: *"When God has begun the work of absolute surrender in you, and when God has accepted your surrender, then God holds Himself bound to care for it and to keep it. Will you believe that?"*

He then goes on to write: *"Oh, we find the Christian life so difficult because we seek for God's blessing while we live in our own will. We should be glad to live the Christian life according to our own liking. We make our own plans and choose our own work, and then we ask the Lord Jesus to come in and take care that sin shall not conquer us too much, and that we shall not go too far wrong; we ask Him to come in and give us so much of His blessing. But our relationship to Jesus ought to be such that we are entirely at His disposal, and every day come to Him humbly and straightforwardly and say: "Lord, is there anything in me that is not according to Thy will, that has not been ordered by You, or that is not entirely given up to You?" Oh, if we would wait and wait patiently, I tell you what the result would be. There would spring up a relationship between us and Christ so close and so tender that we should afterward be amazed at how we formerly could have lived with the idea: "I am surrendered to Christ." We should feel how far distant our intercourse with Him had previously been, and that He can, and does indeed, come and take actual possession of us, and gives unbroken fellowship all the day. The branch calls us to absolute surrender."*

So what does all this mean?

When we *truly* love God and have a true desire to live a Christian life, when we have truly surrendered all to God that He will care for our each and every need, when we come to God daily and pray - yes, earnestly pray - that we would have the fortitude and trust to surrender *all* worries, work, racing thoughts, lack of time, stress, pressure, scarcity and doubt upon Him, then we will stay in bed to greet God each morning and read that Bible not because we have to, but because every last shred of our being *wants* to and *loves* to.

So I pray each day that as I grow in grace and grow in God that He would make every morning in bed reading the Bible something I look forward to just as much as a juicy ribeye steak, a glorious sip of a fine bordeaux, a beautiful hike with my family, a luxurious date with my wife, or a game of tennis at the park.

How about you? Do you ever ponder the absolute power of God, and the near overwhelming privilege of being able to converse and be in union with an almighty Creator of the universe each day? Are you blown away by His simultaneous dangerousness and love? What have you found that enables your daily "woked-ness" to include a deep daily connection with God first thing in the day? As you dwell upon these important questions, it's also of utmost importance to dwell upon your own mortality, as your physical body will fade away, but the soul will go on to exist forever in eternity. So in the final two chapters of Fit Soul, I will present to you important considerations regarding your own passing away from this physical world of flesh into the eternal world of spirit.

For resources, references, links and additional reading and listening material for this chapter, visit FitSoulBook.com/Chapter19.

To Die Is Gain

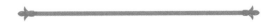

In Chapter 3, I described palliative care practitioner Bronnie Ware's article "Regrets Of The Dying", which is also now more detailed in the recently published book *Top Five Regrets of the Dying: A Life Transformed by the Dearly Departing*. It's worth a read.

In a nutshell, as Bronnie describes, the five regrets most often uttered by those on their deathbed are as follows:

- *I wish I'd had the courage to live a life true to myself, not the life others expected of me.*

- *I wish I hadn't worked so hard.*

- *I wish I'd had the courage to express my feelings.*

- *I wish I had stayed in touch with my friends.*

- *I wish that I had let myself be happier.*

So if you were to act upon these regretful reflections, and if you don't want to die with a lot of regrets, you should:

- *Live a life that's true to who you are, and not driven by who you think the world wants you to be. In other words, be authentic.*

- *Don't spend so much time working. Even if your work is or feels noble and laudable, or even if you're so self-actualized it feels like relaxing play, you may still want to step back and ask yourself how often you use work as an "escape," or to simply immerse yourself in more of the doing that takes you away from being.*

- *Express your feelings. Are you in love? Tell him or her. Are you angry? Speak up (and definitely do not, as I warn in Chapter 14, bury it). Are you lonely? Tell someone. Do you disagree wholeheartedly? Quit being such a people-pleaser or a coward, be bold, and voice your disagreement. You get the idea. Don't cruise through life, stone-faced and so "resilient" that you cannot, will not, fear, or are not vulnerable enough to express your true feelings and emotions.*

- *Keep in touch with your friends (and, dare I say, venture out to make new ones too). I tell you how and why in Chapter 3.*

- *Choose to be happy no matter your circumstances. Stuck on the runway at an airport? Close your eyes, breathe, smile, and finally listen to that Spotify music playlist you've been too busy to savor. Waiting in line at the grocery store when you're late for an appointment? It's not worth fretting. You don't have control. Use it as a much-needed opportunity to stretch, read a few pages on your smartphone's Kindle, or listen to a few minutes of a podcast. At a boring dinner party? Quit sighing with discontent and instead tell your favorite joke from sixth grade to lighten the mood, or ask everybody which superhero they want to be for the night. You get the idea. Be that person who is peaceful, calm, and radiates joy.*

Of course, there are plenty of other "tips" one can find when it comes to dying with no regrets. For example, two of my favorite such resources of late are the article "Die With No Regrets: Follow These 43 Life Lessons" and the book *Don't Waste Your Life*, by John Piper, both of which I'll link to on the resources page for this chapter.

But recently, as I was reading Philippians 1:21 in the Bible, I came across and had a chance to ponder Apostle Paul's words: *"For to me, to live is Christ and to die is gain."*

To die is *gain*?

In other words, one could think of their death on an even more meaningful level than simply dying with "no regrets?" One could experience death as something just as meaningful as life? One could consider and plan for their death to be an event that may very well indeed rock the planet and change the world?

Let's explore that intriguing concept, shall we?

WHAT DOES DYING TO GAIN MEAN?

To understand Paul's words, I think we must first look at the context of his statement *"to die is gain"*.

Up to this time, Paul had suffered much in his missionary journeys. He had been beaten, stoned, hated, mocked, shipwrecked, snake-bitten and, at the time of the writing, was imprisoned. But yet he seemed to find a strange joy in each of these afflictions, because each trial strengthened his faith in leaps and bounds, and allowed him to become an even stronger missionary and champion for Christ. In other passages of Scripture, he describes how he considers his body "as a living sacrifice" (Romans 12:1). for God's kingdom, and also says that because he had faithfully run the race set before him (Hebrews 12:1), he knew God would be honored not only during his life but also at his death (Philippians 1:19–20). He lived a life of great sacrifice and love for others and therefore was assured that even his death would glorify God in a magnificent way.

He would inspire.

He would be remembered.

The seeds of love he had planted across the Mediterranean and beyond would go on to touch the lives of many, and exponentially increase the knowledge of the Hero's Journey of Jesus, far beyond what he would ever have been able to accomplish as one man during one short life.

Paul knew that heaven would be far better than his earthly life, and that in heaven he would be present with God in a place devoid of sin, sickness, and death (2 Corinthians 5:8). But he also knew that before that time came, his purpose on Earth was to live as a beacon light of hope in a world plagued with the darkness of sin and death (Matthew 5:16).

So how can we do this too?

How can we live our own lives so that our death is also gain?

3 WAYS TO LIVE YOUR LIFE SO THAT YOUR DEATH IS GAIN

I think there are three ways to live your life so that your death is gain. I've discovered great meaning and peace from incorporating each of these concepts into my own life, and wish I had taken each of these steps much earlier in my life (as is a repeated theme in this book, not with regret, but only with gratefulness for the road that brought me to where I am thus far). But no matter your age, and no matter how close you suspect you may be to your own death, it is never too late to start.

Here is how you can begin:

1. Possess a purpose statement that loves God and loves others.

Identify your purpose in life and enable yourself to achieve that unique purpose to the very best of your ability while loving God and loving others as fully as possible with that purpose.

See, true and lasting happiness is not achieved by external circumstances, not your thoughts, not your intentions, not even your feelings, but your inner soul. In his book *Soul Keeping,* author John Ortberg defines the soul as that aspect of your whole being that correlates, integrates and enlivens everything else. He writes that we all have two worlds: an outer world that is visible and public and obvious, and an inner world that may be chaotic and dark, or may be gloriously beautiful.

In the end, the outer world fades, and all you are left with then is your inner world.

But ironically, the more obsessed we are with ourselves, our fitness, our cognitive performance, our finances, and our food, the more we tend to neglect our souls. When your soul is not centered and right, you tend to define yourself by your accomplishments, your physical appearance, your title, or your social circles and friends. But then, when you lose these, you tend to lose your identity. I've experienced this myself when I've gotten injured, sick, or had a poor race or workout and subsequently felt like I was losing my happiness and transitioning to a lower level of energy vibration because I was losing my identity as an athlete or a healthy person. Suddenly the emptiness of those shallow pursuits becomes distinctly magnified. Perhaps this is why one of my favorite Bible verses, Mark 8:36 says, *"What does it profit a man to gain the whole world and forfeit his soul?"*

So *how* do you connect with and care for your soul?

You must ask yourself: what is the core part of you that you want folks to talk about at your funeral?

In other words, what is your life's *purpose*?

I tell you in great detail in Chapter 8. Go read it and follow all the instructions. This is important. Set a time to complete the assignment in that chapter and challenge yourself within a month's time to have your single, succinct purpose statement memorized. Then, as I teach you in Chapter 10, revisit that purpose statement every evening.

2. Be humble and meek.

As paradoxical as it may seem, for your death to rock this planet and for your greatness to be fondly remembered, you should live your life in a spirit of meek, humble service towards your fellow human. Jesus said, *"Blessed are the meek, for they shall inherit the earth"* (Matthew 5:5).

Yet meekness and humility is not celebrated in our day and age. Instead, we are surrounded by modern pop culture and entertainment that teaches us that to truly become great and be remembered, we must do the exact opposite. We must become rich and powerful. We must hustle day and night like media mogul Gary Vaynerchuk. We must be aggressive in business and self-promotional in marketing. We must crush others on our rise to the top. We must paint ourselves as living lives of unreachable perfection on our social media channels. We must show no signs of weakness or vulnerability. If we don't amass massive homes, piles of cash, a well-balanced portfolio, and a C-suite executive position in a successful company, then we are unlikely to be remembered for long after we pass, right? Therefore, we must all strive to be great kings and queens.

So in our fallen world, humility is often correlated to weakness. But being meek and humble does not mean you must be weak, tame, or lacking in courage. It simply means that you refuse to inflate your own self-estimation or think more highly of yourself than you ought to think. To be meek is to accept your strengths and limitations for what they truly are, instead of constantly trying to portray yourself in the best possible light. By recognizing our true strengths and weaknesses, we can not only find peace by living realistically, but we can also find the humility that allows us to serve others in a meaningful way, with no judgement, no shaming, and no thought of our own gain.

Harold Bingham Lee, an American religious leader and educator, summarized meekness excellently when he wrote:

> "A meek man is defined as one who is not easily provoked or irritated and forbearing under injury or annoyance. Meekness is not synonymous with weakness. The meek man is the strong, the mighty, the man of complete self-mastery. He is the one who has the courage of his moral convictions, despite . . . pressure. . . . In controversy his judgment is the court of last resort, and his sobered counsel quells the rashness of the mob. He is humble-minded; he does not bluster. . . . He is a natural leader and is the chosen of army and navy, business and church to lead where other men follow. He is the 'salt' of the earth and shall inherit it."

That kind of meek human is who we should strive to be.

After all, Jesus - the greatest King who ever lived - washed his disciples feet. **Will you do the same for those in your life? Or will you strive so hard to "be remembered" that you wind up rich and successful, but lonely and possibly even despised?**

As you consider the answer to those questions, I would encourage you to go watch Michael Jordan's retirement speech, which I'll link to on the resources page for this chapter. Jordan was one of the greatest basketball players that ever lived, right? Yet if you watch his speech, you'll see a slightly sad and unfulfilled individual still seeming to teem with angst, excessive pride and bitterness.

In the years after Michael's retirement, his rise to greatness in basketball became marred with stories of how how he punched a teammate in the face during a practice, how he belittled less-talented peers, how he was fueled by a ruthless anger and bitterness, and how his competitiveness on the golf course, gambling, or in any other competitive venue resulted in many beginning to remember him not for his greatness, but for his divisiveness and rage. This is a perfect example of how pride and superiority, at first, may seem like greatness, but in the end, results in the world instead remembering the fierce arrogance that often accompanies a lack of humility in one's "rise to the top".

Trust me: in the end, that's probably not who you want to be.

3. Write your own obituary.

Although it sounds a bit macabre, writing your own obituary can be a powerful exercise to help you clearly identify whether you are, as John Piper writes in his book *Don't Waste Your Life*, wasting your life frittering away in, as Napoleon Hill writes in his book *Outwitting The Devil*, a hypnotic trance of meaningless and less-than-impactful habits, rituals and routines that neither fully serve your purpose nor fully serve your fellow human.

There are plenty of instructions you can find online about how to go about writing your own obituary, but there are no hard-and-fast rules. You can begin by writing whatever comes to mind, even if it feels like a stream of consciousness. As you begin, don't overthink this exercise or excessively edit, censor, analyze, or critique. Use words, phrases, sentences or paragraphs. Schedule a quiet 30-60 minutes to answer questions such as:

- *What and/or who did you impact or change? Why?*

- *What character traits and values did you consistently demonstrate over your life? At your core, who were you?*

- *Who did you care for? How did you impact or change those you cared for?*

- *What did you care about? This also ties deeply into your purpose statement described above.*

- *What did you show interest in? What were you passionate or enthusiastic about?*

- *What were the major accomplishments in your life? At the ages of 20, 30 40, 50, 60, 70, and beyond?*

What kind of legacy did you leave behind? How were your children, other members of your family, or your connections and relationships impacted by your life?

For inspiration, tips, and plenty of examples of good obituaries, I recommend the two online examples I'll link to on the resources page for this chapter. When you're finished writing your obituary, look it over, and ask yourself questions such as:

- *If I died today, would the world be better because of how I had lived?*

- *Do I feel as though I am fully living my purpose with the direction in which my life is headed?*

- *Am I creating a legacy, and if so what is the legacy that I'm creating?*

- *What's missing from my life that would allow me to love God and love others more fully?*

- *What do I need to do in order for my obituary to be "complete?"*

Then, write a second, fantasy obituary in which you write down all of the things you currently wish you had done with your life when you are reading your current obituary. Pay attention to what changes. Then realize that, especially if you're still reading this, then you're probably not dead yet! Begin making any changes that you need to so that you can live so that the second, fantasy obituary becomes a reality.

I've personally found that one of the very best tools for setting you up to create a meaningful obituary is a "Lifebook" course that I completed two years ago. It was one of the most transformative processes I've ever discovered for crystal-clear clarity, purpose, and direction in life. You can listen to an entire podcast I recorded about that experience via a link I'll include on the resources page for this chapter.

These three exercises - intimately knowing and living your purpose statement; living a life steeped in humility and meekness; and writing your own obituary - will not only give you a new perspective on your own death, but ensure that when you do die, your death is gain, and both your life and your death will have impacted the lives of many in an exponentially profound and positive way.

I encourage you to weave these practices not only into your own life but to teach them to your family, too, so that as part of your legacy, your children and your children's children will incorporate them as honorable traditions in your family for years to come (I teach you more about the concept of meaningful traditions in Chapter 5.

Summary

Finally, remember. death is not a loss.

In death, our spirits will be made perfect, we will be free of sin, and we will be finished with the inner war against our flesh that constantly threatens to derail us during our journey in a mortal body (Hebrews 12:22–23). In death, we will be relieved of the pain of this world (Luke 16:24–25) and granted profound, eternal rest and serenity in our souls (Revelation 6:9–11). In death, we will be taken home to live with our Creator, finally cured of the deep homesickness that the whole human race has, even without knowing it (2 Corinthians 5:8). In death, we will get to go and be smiling with our savior Christ, forever (Philippians 1:21–23).

So death is not something you should dread.

You may even subconsciously crave it. Heck, Paul was a man who craved death and alluded to his desire to die. Once more, we can return to the words of Paul, who said in Philippians:

> *"...For me to live is Christ, and to die is gain. If I am to live in the flesh, that means fruitful labor for me. Yet which I shall choose I cannot tell. I am hard-pressed between the two. My desire is to depart and be with Christ, for that is far better."*

See, we each feel a pull of heaven and yearn for an eternal bliss that goes on far after our bodies have exhaled their last breath. This is what C.S. Lewis described as a "God-shaped" hole in our hearts - an endless abyss that we can dump more money and fancy cars and bigger homes and exercise and diet and even noble pursuits such as family and charity into - but an abyss that will never feel complete, satisfying or fulfilling unless we have discovered the deep satisfaction and joy that comes from peaceful union with God.

Augustine also highlighted a similar idea when he famously wrote, *"Thou hast made us for Thyself, and our hearts are restless until they rest in Thee."* and Indian Christian missionary Sadhu Sundar Singh writes in his book *With and Without Christ:* *"In comparison with this big world, the human heart is only a small thing. Though the world is so large, it is utterly unable to satisfy this tiny heart. Man's ever-groaning soul and its capacities can only be satisfied in the infinite God. As water is restless until it reaches its level, so the soul has no peace until it rests in God."*

Perhaps the best summation of this God-shaped hole and the original concept of it can be found in Blaise Pascal's writings *"Pensées"*, which are a series of defenses of the Christian religion. In Pensées, Pascal says:

> *"What else does this craving, and this helplessness, proclaim but that there was once in man a true happiness, of which all that now remains is the empty print and trace? This he tries in vain to fill with everything around him, seeking in things that are not there the help he cannot find in those that are, though none can help, since this infinite abyss can be filled only with an infinite and immutable object; in other words by God himself."*

So while wandering this earth during the short time that we have here, we can find ultimate peace and fulfillment through union with God - which I recommend you pursue through reading the Bible and following the commandments within it, living your life's purpose to the glory of God in full presence and selfless love for others, believing upon the Hero's Journey of Jesus, and incorporating the spiritual disciplines into your life.

But the final lasting peace and bliss will come when we exhale our last breath, having lived a life that truly glorified God, and having prepared to leave this planet a better place than it was when we were born into it. At that point, when we pass, our death can very much be gain.

And on that final exhale, I plan to say, as Jesus and so many other great martyrs and men and women of God that came after him said, "Into Thy hands, I commit my Spirit."

How about you? Will your death rock this planet? Have you written your own obituary? Do you ever think about regrets you may have when on your deathbed? And finally, if you want to gain a positive perspective on what will happen once you do take that final breath, then keep reading, for it is far more thrilling and exciting than you may have even considered!

For resources, references, links and additional reading and listening material for this chapter, visit *FitSoulBook.com/Chapter20*.

A Slice of Heaven

In Chapter 18, I told you that I really don't think God is a nice old man in soft white robes sitting on a cloud and playing a harp.

Neither do I think that Heaven itself will be an experience that is oft-portrayed in pop culture, cartoons, and literature—all of us adorned with halos and angel wings and perched on a fluffy cloud kind of doing...just about nothing (except perhaps, strumming a giant gold harp)...as though we were all eternally stuck on some kind of ethereal desert island. Just Google "Gary Larson Heaven" for a perfect cartoonish portrayal of how most folks these days portray life in eternity (you'll see a lone, bored guy in wings sitting on a cloud, thinking "I wish I'd brought a magazine").

Neither (to use an analogy you psychonauts out there might relate with) do I believe that Heaven will simply be one big long extended and eternal version of a giant blissful hit of DMT, **which is how I've often heard plant medicine enthusiasts describe their notion of Heaven to be.**

Don't get me wrong, as I touch upon in the introductory chapter to this book and as I will repeat here: I certainly think that there is an appropriate, responsible and purposeful use God intended for plant (or synthetic) medicine in the very same way there is an appropriate, responsible and purposeful use for a nice Bordeaux, a touch of tobacco from a cigar or pipe, or a double espresso shot pumpkin spiced latte. For example, I personally derive a great deal of energetic and creative benefit from the left and right merging of the brain hemispheres, the increase in sensory perception, and the neuronal growth that occurs when I microdose with a bit of psilocybin or LSD on a long writing day; the relaxing or the socially and sexually enhancing benefits of a touch of MDMA or cannabis; and even the enormous spectrum of insights and ideas I gain from a more intensive so-called "journey." Plant medicine, when used responsibly, can be a blessing - but, just like alcohol, nicotine, caffeine, St. John's wort or any other popular substance humankind has discovered to adjust dials in the brain - can also be used as an addiction, an escape and a dangerous replacement for God.

But I digress now from my original point...

...which is that I doubt Heaven is going to be an "infinity version" of how you feel when you're just lazing around doing absolutely nothing without a care in the world on a quiet Sunday afternoon. While I certainly acknowledge, as you'll read later, that in Heaven we will indeed experience blissful relaxation beyond our wildest imagination, I also believe we will be in a state in which we are also inspired and enjoy to do other things, like hiking, swimming, playing, creating, socializing, singing and laughing. I actually can't think of anyone - even the busiest and most stressed folks I know - who could just "sit around and do nothing" for any longer than about a month before beginning to go stir crazy.

Author Mark Twain had an astute observation on this topic. Growing up, I loved Twain's novels. I still think he's one of the most talented writers America has ever produced. But despite my love of Twain, he also portrays a similarly boring view of Heaven. In *The Adventures of Huckleberry Finn*, Huck tells the tale of what the widow Miss Watson, who was the strict, old, obnoxious Christian sister of Huck's main guardian, informed him about Heaven:

> *"She went on and told me all about the good place. She said all a body would have to do there was go around all day long with a harp and sing, forever and ever. So I didn't think much of it. . . . I asked her if she reckoned Tom Sawyer would go there, and she said, not by a considerable sight. I was glad about that because I wanted him and me to be together."*

Twain's Huck seemed pretty disappointed (and rightly so) with this pious Christian spinster's view of Heaven. What he really desired a place a boy would love—a place of adventure, meaning, magic, pleasure, and friendship. As Randy Alcorn says in his book *Heaven* (which I highly recommend as an epic read):

> *"If Miss Watson had told Huck what the Bible says about living in a resurrected body and being with people we love on a resurrected Earth with gardens and rivers and mountains and untold adventures—now that would have gotten his attention!"*

John Eldredge, another favorite author of mine, sums the problem with this boring view of Heaven up quite nicely in his book *"The Journey Of Desire"*:

> *"Nearly every Christian I have spoken with has some idea that*

eternity is an unending church service. . . . We have settled on an
image of the never-ending sing-along in the sky, one great hymn
after another, forever and ever, amen. And our heart sinks. Forever
and ever? That's it? That's the good news? And then we sigh and feel
guilty that we are not more 'spiritual.' We lose heart, and we turn
once more to the present to find what life we can."

I wholeheartedly agree with Randy and John. I just really don't see evidence in the Bible that Heaven is going to be like sitting in a stale, regimented church service that seems a bit like a Groundhog Day experience, but for a million, billion, infinity years.

Instead, there are a multitude of epic, thrilling, and blissful experiences I look forward to in Heaven, including:

- *A brand new beautiful and fully restored planet Earth, the way God originally intended it to be, with all masterfully designed flora and fauna co-existed with us humans for all eternity in a garden city of the most exquisite proportions...*

- *Fish, birds, animals, and all living and breathing creatures restored to their perfect state and living in harmony with us...*

- *Heavenly feasts of scrumptious food and mouth-watering drinks beyond our wildest culinary imaginations...*

- *Massive libraries of the greatest books ever written, both new and old, with an eternity of time to read them all...*

- *The greatest collection of instruments the world has ever known and the ability to be able to play them all while singing songs of deep, loving worship to my Creator, forever and ever...*

The list goes on and on and on, ad infinitum. Just read the book *Heaven* if you want a full Biblically-based insider view of all the glorious experiences we'll enjoy in Heaven.

But if you were to put me on the spot today and make me list the top three things I'm most eagerly anticipating in Heaven—and you were to already account for the fact that being able to worship my Creator for the rest of all time was already a "given"— I'd tell you three things, each of which I've chosen because I feel as though I'm already getting a tiny glimpse here on Earth of how glorious the Heavenly version of these three things will be.

So, based on the tiny slice of Heavenly cake I've tasted in my mortal life on a broken Earth thus far, here are the three Heavenly morsels I'm licking my lips over (and pardon the alliteration).

THREE SLICES OF HEAVEN

1. Create

Think about this...

...you and I were made in the image of God (Genesis 1:26-27), and God is the great Creator. Human beings, therefore, dissimilar from all other animals, possess the unique ability to be able to "creatively create." That is, unless you swallow the notorious argument that beavers create masterful dams or a trained elephant with a paintbrush can make a tree shape on a canvas or that a monkey hitting keys at random on a typewriter keyboard for an infinite amount of time will create any given text, such as the complete works of William Shakespeare (just use a search engine to look up the infinite monkey theorem if you are scratching your head).

Here during our finite, broken lives on Earth, we manage to create giant silver tubes that float gracefully through the sky carrying hundreds of humans 40,000 feet above Earth's surface, massive skyscrapers stretching into the clouds with luscious gardens adorned on their rooftops, and tiny, slick boxes we carry in our pockets that carry more information a fingertip's touch away than all the world's grandest ancient and modern libraries combined.

Just imagine being able to similarly create in Heaven, but in a much more expansive and profound way. What masterpieces could you form if you had millions or billions of years on your hands? This doesn't seem silly to me. God created the human constitution with a driven desire to create, experiment, design, manufacture, fashion, fabricate, and formulate (there's that darn alliteration again, sorry!). This isn't some modern evolutionarily acquired trait: archeology constantly reveals that from cave paintings to Stonehenge to the Pyramids, humankind has created from our very beginnings. It's the way God made us and there's no reason to believe he won't continue to take joy and pleasure in our Creation when we are in eternal union with Him in Heaven (which the Bible clearly tells us is actually a "new Heaven and new Earth").

Being able to work on a watercolor art masterpiece for a thousand years, play a guitar until I have the skills of the greatest guitarist our current world has ever known, or design a new spacecraft that can carry me to the moon and beyond gets me pretty excited. Who knows? My passion for creating here on the "old Earth" is just a tiny slice of the creative cake I'll be blessed to consume on the "new Earth." Possessing an infinite and unchained power of Creation is a pretty exciting and stimulating thought, isn't it?

As a quick aside, I encourage you to never underestimate this built-in core desire to create: If you aren't engaged in some type of creative work or hobby now, then I implore you to begin—it feeds the deep-rooted desires of your soul! And what is the opposite of creation? Consumption. Something deep down inside us humans would actually rather learn to craft the perfect piece of sushi instead of binge-watching cooking shows on Netflix, throw a flawless football spiral rather than burning our eyeballs out on a screen for three hours during a Sunday afternoon NFL game, or learn to tell a funny, entertaining joke or story rather than parking ourselves in front of a YouTube stand-up comedy channel, yet our inherent laziness and resistance to the call of creation can often drive us to instead stay stuck in consumption mode.

Take America for example: Once a land of innovation, creativity, and new designs and inventions, we are now severely outpaced by countries such as China in terms of our actual creation and production because we've become a largely consumerist culture, and constant consumption is now considered normal and acceptable. But I guarantee you'll find yourself far more happy and fulfilled if you create more than you consume, every day. The world would be better for it.

2. Calm

In six days, God created the universe in a great display of the most meaningful "work" ever accomplished, then He rested on the seventh day (Genesis 2:2). Throughout the Bible, God shows how much he values rest and relaxation (e.g. Hebrews 4:11 "Make every effort to enter that rest..." or Matthew 11:28 "Come to me all you who are weary, and I will give you rest."), setting aside days and weeks of rest and even resting the entire Earth itself every seventh year (Leviticus 25:4-5 - "...but in the seventh year the land is to have a year of sabbath rest, a sabbath to the Lord. Do not sow your fields or prune your vineyards. Do not reap what grows of itself or harvest the grapes of your untended vines. The land is to have a year of rest.")

The calm feeling that washes over you when you finally lay your head on a pillow after a full day of work, that glass of wine you enjoy on the porch while watching the sunset melt away the stress of the day, or perhaps most meaningfully, the entire day of blissful relaxation, celebration, and fellowship we all have the privilege to enjoy on the Sabbath are all just tiny tastes of the eternal constant and continual calm we will experience in Heaven.

In Heaven, despite our natural desire to creatively create, there will be actually no *need* to work, at least not in the way we think of it here on Earth. Certainly, as sinless humans did in the Garden of Eden, in Heaven we will very likely be gardeners, be caring for animals, be hiking epic mountain ranges, and be enjoying the new Heaven and new Earth in all its glory, but in a manner more like we do here on a relaxed Sunday—wandering out to the backyard garden to pluck a few fresh, ripe tomatoes, bringing our happy dog out for a walk, and taking the family on a long, scenic hike.

So will we "work" in Heaven? It's certainly possible. Work began before sin—shown by the primary intense work of God in creating for six consecutive days. But our work will be different. As Randy Alcorn says in *Heaven*:

> *"What kind of work will we do in Heaven? Maybe you'll build a cabinet with Joseph of Nazareth. Or with Jesus. Maybe you'll tend sheep with David, discuss medicine with Luke, sew with Dorcas, make clothes with Lydia, design a new tent with Paul or Priscilla, write a song with Isaac Watts, ride horses with John Wesley, or sing with Keith Green..."*

We know that when people here on Earth "retire," they often die much sooner. As image-bearers of God the Creator, meaningful work is woven into our DNA. But our work in Heaven will be purely joyful and fulfilling as we engage in the fully self-actualized, pleasurable pursuit of creating.

Just imagine the blissful calm of being able to lay back, interlace your hands behind your head, stare up at the sky, and realize that there's no actual *pressure* to do *anything* besides sing and worship and bask in God's glory while reflecting it back to Him for the rest of all time. No phone calls, no emails, no bills, no traffic, no rushing, and no stress. We get to experience 1/7 of that calm during our lives here on Earth, on each Sunday of the week, but we'll get 7/7 of that same calm, but with many, many upgrades, upon our arrival in Heaven. How peaceful that will be!

3. Connection

Many folks believe that we won't desire or engage in any relationships in Heaven aside from our relationship with God. For example, theologians Augustine and Aquinas both imagined that in Heaven we will focus exclusively on God and that any other relationships or friendships between human beings would be absent or insignificant.

But if, here on the Old Earth, meaningful human connections, beginning with the companionship of Adam and Eve, were assessed by God to take us from "not good" to "very good," why would we expect Him to suddenly change his mind in Heaven and on the New Earth? After all, God designed us to need and depend upon our fellow humans and image-bearers of Him, creating in us a desire to depend not only on our relationship with Him for our ultimate happiness and joy but also our relationship with others. God is a Father and fathers naturally delight in their children's close relationships. God takes pleasure in our families, friendships, and relationships; and there's no reason to believe he won't continue to do so in Heaven.

Even near the end of his life, Augustine himself said:

> *"We have not lost our dear ones who have departed from this life, but have merely sent them ahead of us, so we also shall depart and shall come to that life where they will be more than ever dear as they will be better known to us, and where we shall love them without fear of parting."*

In addition, priest, church historian and orator Venerable Bede wrote of Heaven:

> *"A great multitude of dear ones is there expecting us; a vast and mighty crowd of parents, brothers, and children, secure now of their own safety, anxious yet for our salvation, long that we may come to their right and embrace them, to that joy which will be common to us and to them, to that pleasure expected by our fellow servants as well as ourselves, to that full and perpetual felicity.... If it be a pleasure to go to them, let us eagerly and covetously hasten on our way, that we may soon be with them, and soon be with Christ..."*

English Puritan church leader Richard Baxter wrote:

> *"I know that Christ is all in all; and that it is the presence of God that makes Heaven to be Heaven. But yet it much sweetens the*

thoughts of that place to me that there are such a multitude of my
most dear and precious friends in Christ."

In his book *Heaven: A World Of Love*, **Jonathan Edwards comments that:**

"...every Christian friend that goes before us from this world, is a
ransomed spirit waiting to welcome us in heaven. There will be the
infant of days that we have lost below, through grace to be found
above; there the Christian father, and mother, and wife, and child,
and friend, with whom we shall renew the holy fellowship of the
saints, which was interrupted by death here, but shall be
commenced again in the upper sanctuary, and then shall never end.
There we shall have company with the patriarchs and fathers and
saints of the Old and New Testaments, and those of whom the world
was not worthy, with whom on earth we were only conversant by
faith. And there, above all, we shall enjoy and dwell with God the
Father, whom we have loved with all our hearts on earth; and with
Jesus Christ, our beloved Savior, who has always been to us the
chief among ten thousands, and altogether lovely; and with the
Holy Ghost, our Sanctifier, and Guide, and Comforter; and shall be
filled with all the fullness of the Godhead forever!"

Of course, friendships will be transformed into the pinnacle of perfect glory in
Heaven, with none of the annoying and divisive cliques, exclusiveness, arrogance,
posturing, belittling, and jealousy we currently experience. Instead, we can anticipate
lounging with all our friends, both old and new, at God's great feast for the rest of all
time—laughing, growing, playing, and sharing stories for millions of years, into
eternity. I certainly relish the thought of Heaven not being an isolated experience in
which I'm all by myself on a lonely cloud floating through the sky, but rather a giant
gathering of parties, camaraderie, and joy the likes of which has never before been
seen!

Summary

Of course, as I alluded to earlier, creation, calm, and connection are just a smattering of the smorgasbord of the joy and pleasures we will experience at the right hand of God forevermore. But my taste of the happiness derived from creative expression, a restful Sabbath day, and friendships and relationships here on Old Earth make me savor the ultimate richness of those same experiences I'll get to enjoy in Heaven.

So how about you? Will I share the joys of Heaven with you? Do you long for Heaven in the same way that I do? If you want to know more about how to be welcomed into the loving embrace of Jesus and share in the eternal bliss of Heaven, then read about the Hero's Journey in Chapter 9. You'll discover exactly how.

CONCLUSION

Congratulations. By getting to this final chapter, you have taken a significant journey of spiritual fitness in your path to a fit soul. I trust that within the pages of this book, you have found new inspiration and insight for your health, purpose, presence, life, relationship with others and relationship with God.

So where do you go from here?

First, I encourage you to wake each day and do as extraordinary a job you can with everything that God places upon your plate, trusting Him for direction each day. You may not yet know the exact plan God has for your life, and that's OK. Even the most successful and spiritually fit human beings don't have a complete, crystal clear roadmap for their life magically laid out in front of them. But they do have a sense of purpose, a sense of presence, and an intimate relationship with and trust in their Creator, and a deep desire to glorify God and love others by applying extreme excellence to every last task that is placed in front of them each day. So trust God, work hard, and be extraordinary.

Second, get a good Bible. Splurge on yourself. It is one of the most important decisions you can make. Consider praying and reading your Bible even more than you currently are, constantly seeking direction from God and being in union with Him 24-7 for Him to direct your paths, realizing that he laughs at the plans of humans, but honors those who trusts in His own plans while asking for, seeking and listening to His wisdom and discernment.

If you read Fit Soul, you likely enjoy reading a variety of books. But please understand that the Bible must be the most important book in your library and the foundation of every life plan you make. You must be turning to God's word every day for wisdom, discernment and to reveal to you "the next steps" for your life. The Bible must be the foundational book in your library, and be given a holy place in your household. It is the most powerful and holy weapon God has ever created, and is your source for absolute truth. In the long run, you don't need any other source of wisdom than the Bible.

So I encourage you to place the Bible upon your heart so that you can rely upon it both day and night. It will help you cut through all the darkness and confusion you'll undoubtedly be confronted with as you navigate through life in a fallen and sinful world. When combined with the other spiritual disciplines you find within the pages of *Fit Soul*, you will be equipped to defend yourself against the fiery darts of the evil one and also to make a strong defense for the hope that is within you.

Third, for additional reading and supplementary materials, check out all the resources pages for each chapter in this book, all of which you can find at FitSoulBook.com. Below, I also recommend a few other titles I've personally written that include plenty of spiritual lessons I've learned along my own path in life, along with plenty of additional health, fitness and nutrition advice, including:

- *Beyond Training: Mastering Endurance, Health & Life* at BeyondTrainingBook.com

- *Boundless: Upgrade Your Brain, Optimize Your Body & Defy Aging* at BoundlessBook.com

- *The Boundless Cookbook* at BoundlessCookbook.com

- *The Spiritual Disciplines Journal* at SpiritualDisciplinesJournal.com

Finally, if you found this book inspirational, transformational or in any way helpful, please share it with your friends and family, or on social media, and also visit FitSoulBook.com and use the contact form there to leave me a message, a question, a testimonial or any other encouraging words!

Yours In Christ,

Ben Greenfield
FitSoulBook.com

ABOUT THE COVER

✦━━━━━━━━━━━━━━✦

You may be wondering why I chose to adorn the cover of Fit Soul with an image of a kneeling medieval-esque warrior knight clad in armor.

The answer is simple, and can be found in the words of one of my favorite and incredibly powerful Bible passages - Ephesians 6:10–18:

> *"Finally, be strong in the Lord and in his mighty power. Put on the full armor of God, so that you can take your stand against the devil's schemes.*
>
> *For our struggle is not against flesh and blood, but against the rulers, against the authorities, against the powers of this dark world and against the spiritual forces of evil in the heavenly realms.*
>
> *Therefore, put on the full armor of God, so that when the day of evil comes, you may be able to stand your ground, and after you have done everything, to stand.*
>
> *Stand firm then, with the belt of truth buckled around your waist, with the breastplate of righteousness in place, and with your feet fitted with the readiness that comes from the gospel of peace. In addition to all this, take up the shield of faith, with which you can extinguish all the flaming arrows of the evil one. Take the helmet of salvation and the sword of the Spirit, which is the word of God.*
>
> *And pray in the Spirit on all occasions with all kinds of prayers and requests. With this in mind, be alert and always keep on praying for all the Lord's people."*

If you're handy at math, then you counted seven distinct pieces of spiritual armor listed in the passage above that can equip you to be strong in the Lord and His mighty power. When I'm spiritually struggling, know that I'm entering into a situation in which I will encounter significant temptations, or am about to embark on travel away from my family and Christian support network, I often imagine adorning myself with each of these seven pieces of armor, specifically:

1. The Belt of Truth

A soldier must be girded with a belt, which in the time the passage above was written was made of metal and thick heavy leather and served as the carrying place for a Roman soldier's sword. The belt also had an armored section in the front to protect the vitals, and helped to hold all other pieces of the armor together. Truth is a belt that holds your spiritual armor together as well. As you learn in Fit Soul, absolute truth can be found in the Bible, and you must immerse yourself daily in this truth to be able to protect your spiritual self. So know your Bible, think of it as your belt, and gird yourself up with it.

2. Breastplate of Righteousness

A breastplate protects the vital organs during the heat of the battle, especially when a soldier may not be quick enough to hold up their shield. It was designed for fast and unanticipated advances of the enemy. Living a righteous life - not by our own works - but through the righteousness granted to us by Christ is a powerful way to protect our heart and keep our enemy from successfully striking when we don't expect it. Righteousness means being made right, and includes daily confessions of our sin and laying our burdens at the foot of the cross so that we can enter our spiritual battles with purity of heart.

3. Feet fitted with the Gospel of Peace

In Roman times, a soldier was fitted with sandals that had extremely thick soles to protect the feet from blistering during long marches into battle, and spikes to help the soldier stand firm during battle. Our own protection and firm foundation through the journey of life is the Gospel: Jesus' deity, death, burial and resurrection. As we walk into battle, we possess the hope and deep internal peace that because of His sacrifice and our belief in Him, we shall not perish but have eternal life. Studying and sharing the Gospel and being prepared to defend the hope that is within us will help to build this peace, protection, and firm foundation.

4. Shield of Faith

A shield serves as a soldier's primary defensive weapon. A Roman soldier's shield was made of dense, solid wood, leather, canvas, and metal, and was often doused in water to create a heavy, wet hide that could extinguish the fiery arrows of the enemy. Our own impenetrable shield is faith: a deep trust in God's power and protection, and a confidence knowing that God will hold true to His promises even when the battle is raging as fiercely as ever. In addition, shields used on the field of battle are even stronger when linked with one another, and so, in addition to equipping ourselves with faith and trust in God, we must also band together with fellow believers in churches, small groups and other forms of fellowship to buttress ourselves even more securely against the attacks of the enemy.

5. Helmet of Salvation

A good helmet would cover the most vulnerable areas of a soldier's body: the entire head, face and even between the eyes. Without a helmet, one blow to a soldier's head would almost certainly prove debilitating or fatal, making the rest of the armor completely useless without that helmet. Our helmet of salvation and anointing with the Holy Spirit is therefore critical to our own battle armor. When we know beyond a shadow of a doubt that we are going on to heaven and eternal bliss because of what Christ accomplished on the cross, not even death can defeat us. Without the helmet of salvation, our armor is for naught and there is no victory, but when we don our helmet and stand upon the conviction of our deliverance by Jesus, then we know that, as Romans 8 says, "neither death nor life, neither angels nor principalities, neither the present nor the future, nor any powers, neither height nor depth, nor anything else in all creation, will be able to separate us from the love of God that is in Christ Jesus our Lord".

6. Sword of the Spirit

You may have noticed that the first five pieces of the soldier's arsenal that you have been reading about are all defensive weapons, but this is the first part of the passage in Ephesians in which an offensive weapon is described: the sword. In the hands of a skilled warrior, a sword was considered a deadly weapon that could pierce through even the strongest armor. The sword of the spirit is described as the word of God, which we know from the Bible is sharper than any double edged physical sword. As I have already mentioned, to wield this weapon effectively, you must daily immerse yourself in Scripture, not only reading it, hearing it, singing it, and meditating upon it, but also memorizing it so that in times of battle you have specific verses from the Bible that you can draw upon to resist temptation and fight evil. Jesus relied upon Scripture to defeat Satan when He was tempted in the desert, and we must do the same if we are to yield the greatest offensive weapon against evil that God has ever blessed us with.

7. Prayer

You may have noticed that on the cover of this book, the warrior is kneeling. That is intentional. Although often forgotten or not mentioned as a crucial part of this section of Ephesians, prayer is essential, because without God's union and presence, we are powerless in battle. So we must "fight from our knees," thus blanketing ourselves with His presence that we have prayed upon our bodies, our soul, and our entire spiritual armor. We must be in a daily constancy of prayer, continually connected to God from the time that we wake to the time that we go to sleep. It is such a wonderful blessing that we can speak to the Almighty Creator at any time during the day, and we must make a habit of doing so if we are to be able to resist the daily battles that we will inevitably face. Wake and pray, walk and pray, eat and pray, breathe and pray, pray whenever God has granted you a silent moment during the day, and pray "on all occasions." Make prayer a natural and continual part of your life, so that you are never venturing into battle without the powerful presence of God.

My friends, the war has been won. Jesus accomplished that on the cross. But the daily battle must still be fought. Armed with the defenses and weapons above, you will have all the tools that you need - by the blood of Jesus, the anointing of the Holy Spirit and the grace of God - to enter into that battle with your spirit fully protected.